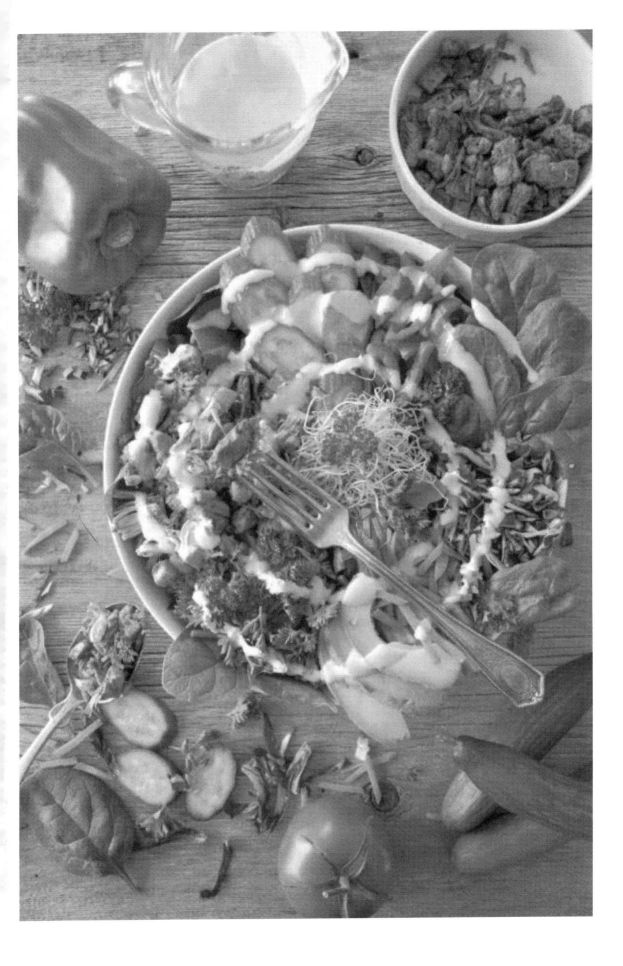

Keto for Cancer Cookbook

1500 Days of Nutritional Facts, Strategies, Ketogenic Recipes, And A Healthy Meal Plan for A Metabolic Approach to Fighting Cancer with Nontoxic Therapies

Dr. Isabelle Monroe

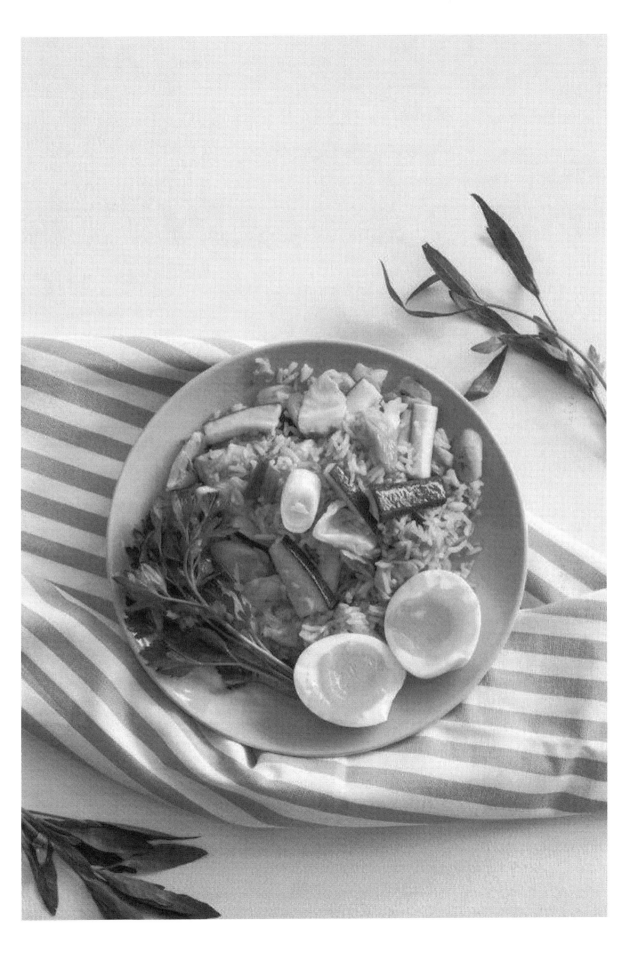

Content

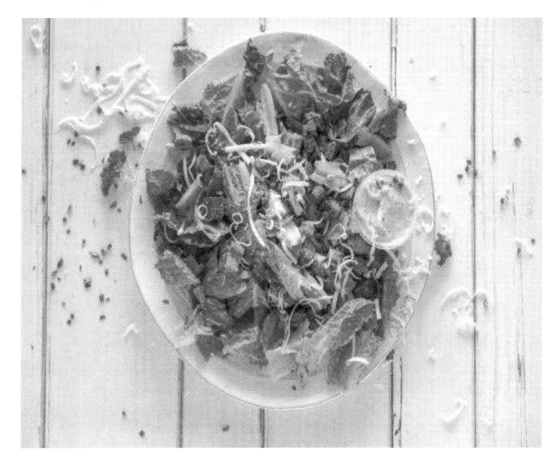

INTRODUCTION

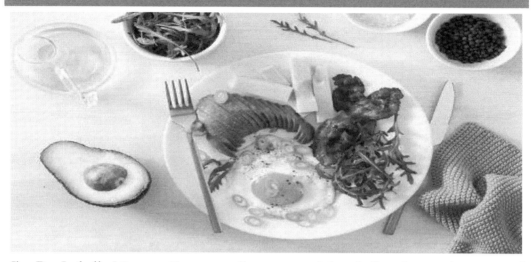

I'm Dr. Isabelle Monroe. For years, I've managed the challenging environment of oncology, watching the sheer tenacity and courage of my patients fighting cancer. Every trip was unique, each story intriguing, but there was a unifying factor - the dogged search of a solution, a light of hope, in the fight against this powerful foe.

The quest to help my patients wasn't a linear road. I scoured through countless resources, studied thoroughly, and tried numerous methods. Through the ups and downs, the successes and setbacks, I became personally familiar with the anger and helplessness that often follow a cancer diagnosis. Yet, in the middle of this struggle, came a glimmer of hope – the ketogenic diet.

The ketogenic diet is not just a dietary choice; it's a metabolic method that uses the power of nutrition in ways that continue to surprise the medical community. Its effect on cancer metabolism and cell processes has been a surprise. The road to discover this potential wasn't easy, but the understanding that the ketogenic diet could be a key player in the fight against cancer was a turning point in my approach to patient care.

As I pen down this cookbook, my heart swells with the hope that it may reach corners of the world where people, families, and caregivers deal with the weight of a cancer diagnosis. The thought that this guide could be a beacon, a roadmap through the confusing maze of dietary choices and medical challenges, brings a deep sense of purpose.

I'm sure, deeply so, that the recipes, nutritional insights, and advice within these pages can be a game-changer. The meticulous selection of ingredients, the thoughtful building of meal plans, and the comprehensive approach to handling the challenges that cancer brings – it's all here to serve as a steadfast partner in your battle against this disease.

Every word, every recipe, every idea is based in the belief that a balanced, nutritionally-focused approach, especially through the ketogenic diet, can offer significant support in controlling and fighting cancer.

So, to each person reading these pages, I offer not just a collection of recipes but a hand to hold, a voice to guide, and a source of constant support. Together, let's start on this journey towards health and energy. Your resolve, combined with the insights shared here, is a strong combo that can indeed beat the challenges posed by cancer.

With sincere wishes for your health and well-being,

WHAT IS THE KETOGENIC DIET?

The ketogenic diet is a very low-carbohydrate, high-fat diet that shares many similarities with the Atkins and low-carb diets. It involves drastically reducing carbohydrate intake and replacing it with fat. This reduction in carbs puts your body into a metabolic state called ketosis.

When you eat a lot of carbohydrates, your body converts them into glucose, which is your body's main source of energy. However, when you restrict your carbohydrate intake, your body instead breaks down stored fat into molecules called ketones for energy.

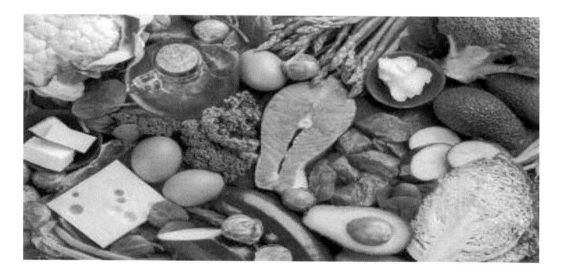

HOW DOES THE KETOGENIC DIET WORK AGAINST CANCER?

There are a number of ways in which the ketogenic diet may help to fight cancer.

- It can starve cancer cells. Cancer cells are more dependent on glucose for energy than normal cells. By restricting carbohydrates, the ketogenic diet can help to starve cancer cells of the fuel they need to grow and survive.

- It can make cancer cells more sensitive to chemotherapy and radiation therapy. Research has shown that the ketogenic diet can make cancer cells more vulnerable to the effects of chemotherapy and radiation therapy. This is because the ketogenic diet can increase the production of reactive oxygen species (ROS), which are molecules that can damage cancer cells.

- It can reduce inflammation. Inflammation is a major driver of cancer development and progression. The ketogenic diet has been shown to reduce inflammation throughout the body.

BENEFITS OF THE KETOGENIC DIET FOR CANCER PATIENTS

In addition to its potential anti-cancer effects, the ketogenic diet can also offer a number of other benefits for cancer patients, including:

- Weight loss. The ketogenic diet is very effective for weight loss, which can be important for cancer patients who are overweight or obese. Excess weight can increase the risk of cancer recurrence and death, so losing weight can improve outcomes.

- Improved insulin sensitivity. The ketogenic diet can help to improve insulin sensitivity, which can be beneficial for cancer patients with diabetes or prediabetes.

- Reduced side effects of cancer treatment. The ketogenic diet may help to reduce some of the side effects of cancer treatment, such as nausea, vomiting, and fatigue.

HOW TO FOLLOW THE KETOGENIC DIET SAFELY AND EFFECTIVELY?

If you are considering following the ketogenic diet, it is important to talk to your doctor first, especially if you have any underlying health conditions.

To follow the ketogenic diet, you will need to restrict your carbohydrate intake to 20-50 grams per day. This means avoiding sugary foods, starchy vegetables, and grains. Instead, you will focus on eating high-fat, low-carbohydrate foods, such as meat, fish, eggs, nuts, seeds, and non-starchy vegetables.

Here are some tips for following the ketogenic diet safely and effectively:

- Eat plenty of non-starchy vegetables. Non-starchy vegetables are low in carbohydrates and high in nutrients. They are also a good source of fiber, which can help to keep you feeling full.

- Choose healthy fats. Not all fats are created equal. Some fats, such as saturated and trans fats, can raise your cholesterol levels and increase your risk of heart disease. Instead, focus on eating healthy fats, such as those found in avocados, olive oil, nuts, and seeds.

- Get enough protein. Protein is essential for building and repairing tissues. When following the ketogenic diet, it is important to make sure that you are getting enough protein. Good sources of protein include meat, fish, eggs, and dairy products.

- Stay hydrated. It is important to stay hydrated when following the ketogenic diet. This is because the ketogenic diet can cause you to lose more fluids through urination. Drink plenty of water throughout the day.

- Monitor your electrolytes. Electrolytes are minerals that are essential for many bodily functions. When following the ketogenic diet, it is important to monitor your electrolyte levels and make sure that you are getting enough. Good sources of electrolytes include sodium, potassium, and magnesium.

It is also important to note that the ketogenic diet is not for everyone. The ketogenic diet can be difficult to follow, and it can cause some side effects, such as fatigue, nausea, and vomiting. If you experience any side effects, talk to your doctor.

The ketogenic diet is a very low-carbohydrate, high-fat diet that has been shown to have a number of potential health benefits, including anti-cancer effects. If you are considering following the ketogenic diet, it is important to talk to your doctor first to make sure that it is safe for you.

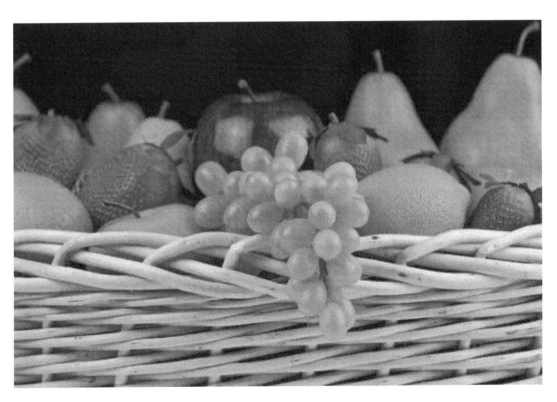

GETTING STARTED ON THE KETO DIET

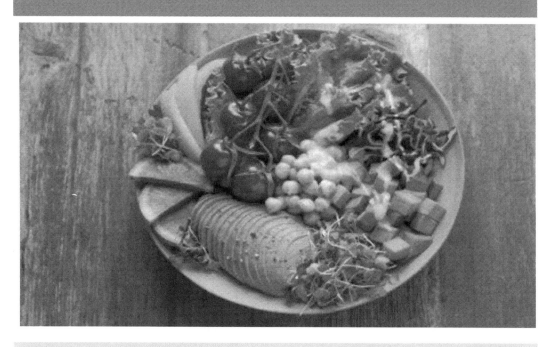

CALCULATING YOUR MACROS

The first step in getting started on the keto diet is to calculate your macros. Macros are the macronutrients that make up your diet: protein, fat, and carbohydrates. On the keto diet, you will need to limit your carbohydrate intake to 20-50 grams per day, and increase your fat intake.

To calculate your macros, you can use an online macro calculator. These calculators will take into account your age, sex, weight, height, and activity level to determine the number of calories and macros you need to consume each day.

Once you have calculated your macros, you need to divide them up into three meals and two snacks. A good starting point is to aim for 30% protein, 50% fat, and 20% carbohydrates.

MEAL PLANNING AND PREPPING

Meal planning and prepping are essential for success on the keto diet. This is because it can be difficult to find keto-friendly options when eating out, and it is important to have healthy meals and snacks on hand at all times.

When meal planning, start by making a list of all the keto-friendly foods you enjoy. Then, create a meal plan that includes a variety of foods from all food groups. It is also important to make sure that your meals are balanced and provide you with all the nutrients you need.

Meal prepping can save you time and hassle throughout the week. Simply cook your meals in advance and portion them out into containers. This will make it easy to grab a healthy meal or snack on the go.

KETO-FRIENDLY FOODS AND INGREDIENTS

The ketogenic diet primarily focuses on low-carbohydrate, high-fat foods. Incorporating the following keto-friendly foods and ingredients is essential for maintaining ketosis and deriving health benefits:

Healthy Fats:

1. **Avocados:** Rich in healthy fats and fiber, making them an ideal keto staple.

2. **Coconut Oil:** A source of medium-chain triglycerides (MCTs), aiding in ketone production.

3. **Olive Oil:** High in monounsaturated fats, offering a healthy option for cooking and dressings.

4. **Nuts and Seeds:** Almonds, walnuts, chia seeds, flaxseeds, and pumpkin seeds provide healthy fats, fiber, and protein.

5. **Fatty Fish:** Salmon, mackerel, and sardines are rich in omega-3 fatty acids.

Low-Carb Vegetables:

1. **Leafy Greens:** Spinach, kale, and Swiss chard are nutrient-dense and low in carbohydrates.

2. **Cruciferous Vegetables:** Broccoli, cauliflower, and Brussels sprouts are high in fiber and low in carbs.

3. **Zucchini:** Versatile and low in carbs, suitable for noodles or as a base for various dishes.

4. **Bell Peppers:** Low in carbohydrates and high in vitamin C.

Protein Sources:

1. **Poultry:** Chicken, turkey, and duck are excellent low-carb protein sources.

2. **Grass-Fed Beef:** A source of protein and healthy fats.

3. **Eggs:** A complete protein and a versatile ingredient for various keto-friendly dishes.

4. **Seafood:** Shrimp, shellfish, and various fish are low in carbs and high in quality protein.

Dairy:

1. **Cheese:** Varieties like cheddar, mozzarella, and cream cheese are low in carbs and rich in fats and protein.

2. **Greek Yogurt:** Opt for full-fat, unsweetened Greek yogurt for a lower carb content.

3. **Heavy Cream:** Useful for adding richness to dishes and beverages.

Condiments and Flavor Enhancers:

1. **Herbs and Spices:** Including basil, oregano, thyme, and cumin to add flavor without adding carbs.

2. **Low-Carb Sauces:** Sugar-free tomato sauce, mayonnaise, and mustard are keto-friendly options.

3. **Stevia or Erythritol:** Natural sweeteners with minimal impact on blood sugar levels.

Beverages:

1. **Water:** Essential for staying hydrated and maintaining overall health.

2. **Coffee and Tea:** Black coffee and unsweetened teas are suitable keto-friendly beverages.

3. **Bone Broth:** Rich in nutrients and collagen, supporting overall health.

Snacks and Treats:

1. **Pork Rinds:** A crunchy, low-carb snack option.

2. **Dark Chocolate:** Opt for high-cocoa content, low-sugar chocolate as an occasional treat.

3. **Keto-friendly Bars:** Look for bars with low net carbs and high fat content.

Avoiding Common Keto Pitfalls

There are a few common keto pitfalls that you should be aware of. Here are some tips to help you avoid them:

- Not eating enough fat: It is important to make sure that you are eating enough fat on the keto diet. This will help you stay in ketosis and avoid hunger pangs.

- Eating too many carbohydrates: It is important to limit your carbohydrate intake to 20-50 grams per day. This can be difficult, but it is essential for success on the keto diet.

- Not drinking enough fluids: It is important to stay hydrated on the keto diet. Drink plenty of water, unsweetened tea, and coffee throughout the day.

- Not getting enough electrolytes: Electrolytes are important for maintaining hydration and muscle function. Make sure to consume enough sodium, potassium, and magnesium on the keto diet.

If you experience any negative side effects while on the keto diet, such as fatigue, headache, or muscle cramps, be sure to talk to your doctor.

Getting started on the keto diet can be daunting, but it does not have to be. By following the tips above, you can make the transition to keto smooth and successful.

BREAKFAST RECIPES

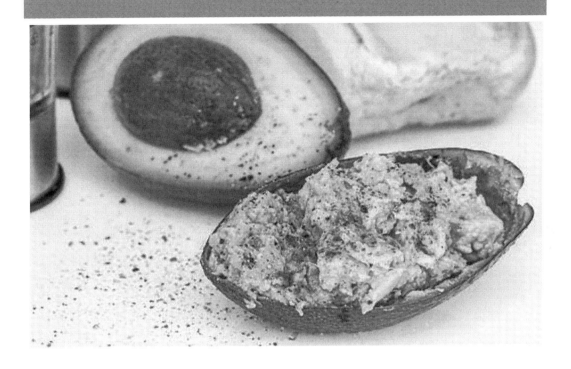

Recipe 1: Keto Avocado Egg Breakfast

Ingredients:

- 2 ripe avocados
- 4 eggs
- Salt and pepper to taste
- Fresh herbs (optional)

Instructions:

1. Preheat the oven to 425°F (220°C).

2. Cut avocados in half and remove pits.

3. Scoop out a little extra avocado to create more space for the egg.

4. Crack an egg into each avocado half.

5. Season with salt and pepper.

6. Place on a baking sheet and bake for 15-20 minutes or until the eggs set.

7. Garnish with fresh herbs if desired.

Meal Prep: Quick and easy, prepare within 30 minutes.

Time: 20 minutes

Nutritional Information:

- Calories: 320

- Protein: 12g

- Fat: 26g

- Carbohydrates: 12g

- Fiber: 9g

Recipe 2: Keto Coconut Chia Pudding

Ingredients:

- 1/4 cup chia seeds

- 1 cup coconut milk

- 1 tsp vanilla extract

- 1 tbsp low-carb sweetener (Stevia or erythritol)

Instructions:

1. Mix chia seeds, coconut milk, vanilla extract, and sweetener in a bowl.

2. Stir well and let it sit for 10 minutes.

3. Stir again to prevent clumping.

4. Cover and refrigerate overnight or for at least 4 hours.

5. Serve with toppings like berries or nuts.

Meal Prep: Prepare the night before for a quick morning meal.

Time: 5 minutes (plus overnight refrigeration)

Nutritional Information:

- Calories: 180

- Protein: 4g

- Fat: 15g

- Carbohydrates: 8g

- Fiber: 6g

Recipe 3: Keto Bacon and Spinach Egg Muffins

Ingredients:

- 6 eggs

- 6 slices bacon, cooked and crumbled

- 1 cup chopped spinach

- Salt and pepper to taste

- 1/2 cup shredded cheese (optional)

Instructions:

1. Preheat oven to 350°F (175°C).

2. Grease a muffin tin.

3. Whisk eggs in a bowl, add bacon, spinach, salt, and pepper.

4. Pour the mixture into the muffin tin, filling each cup about 3/4 full.

5. Sprinkle cheese on top if desired.

6. Bake for 15-20 minutes until set.

7. Allow to cool before removing from the tin.

Meal Prep: Make a batch for the week, reheat as needed.

Time: 30 minutes

Nutritional Information:

- Calories: 220

- Protein: 14g

- Fat: 16g

- Carbohydrates: 2g

- Fiber: 1g

Recipe 4: Keto Zucchini Pancakes

Ingredients:

- 2 cups shredded zucchini
- 2 eggs
- 1/4 cup almond flour
- 1/4 cup grated parmesan cheese
- 1/2 tsp garlic powder
- Salt and pepper to taste
- Olive oil for cooking

Instructions:

1. Place shredded zucchini in a clean kitchen towel and squeeze out excess moisture.

2. In a bowl, combine zucchini, eggs, almond flour, parmesan, garlic powder, salt, and pepper.

3. Heat olive oil in a skillet over medium heat.

4. Scoop 1/4 cup of the mixture onto the skillet, flatten and cook for 3-4 minutes on each side until golden brown.

5. Repeat with the remaining mixture.

Meal Prep: Prepare a large batch and freeze for later use.

Time: 25 minutes

Nutritional Information:

- Calories: 180
- Protein: 10g
- Fat: 12g
- Carbohydrates: 6g
- Fiber: 2g

Recipe 5: Keto Smoked Salmon Roll-Ups

Ingredients:

- 4 oz smoked salmon
- 4 oz cream cheese

- 1 tbsp capers (optional)
- 1 tbsp chopped chives

Instructions:

1. Lay out smoked salmon slices.

2. Spread a thin layer of cream cheese on each slice.

3. Sprinkle capers and chopped chives.

4. Roll up the slices and slice into smaller rolls if desired.

Meal Prep: Quick and convenient, prepare in 10 minutes.

Time: 10 minutes

Nutritional Information:

- Calories: 220
- Protein: 15g
- Fat: 16g
- Carbohydrates: 2g
- Fiber: 0g

Recipe 6: Keto Cauliflower Hash Browns

Ingredients:

- 2 cups riced cauliflower
- 1 egg
- 1/4 cup shredded cheese
- 1/4 tsp garlic powder
- Salt and pepper to taste
- Olive oil for cooking

Instructions:

1. Mix riced cauliflower, egg, shredded cheese, garlic powder, salt, and pepper in a bowl.

2. Heat olive oil in a skillet over medium heat.

3. Form small patties from the mixture and place in the skillet.

4. Cook for 3-4 minutes on each side until golden brown.

Meal Prep: Cook a large batch and refrigerate for quick reheating.

Time: 20 minutes

Nutritional Information:

- Calories: 160

- Protein: 9g

- Fat: 10g

- Carbohydrates: 6g

- Fiber: 3g

Recipe 7: Keto Blueberry Almond Smoothie

Ingredients:

- 1/2 cup frozen blueberries

- 1 cup unsweetened almond milk

- 2 tbsp almond butter

- 1 scoop vanilla protein powder (optional)

- 1 tsp chia seeds (optional)

Instructions:

1. Blend all ingredients until smooth.

2. Add more almond milk if needed for desired consistency.

3. Serve immediately.

Meal Prep: Quick to make, perfect for a busy morning.

Time: 5 minutes

Nutritional Information:

- Calories: 250

- Protein: 12g

- Fat: 18g

- Carbohydrates: 14g

- Fiber: 6g

Recipe 8: Keto Breakfast Burrito Bowl

Ingredients:

- 4 slices bacon, chopped

- 4 eggs

- 1/2 avocado, sliced

- 1/4 cup shredded cheese

- Salsa (optional)

- Salt and pepper to taste

Instructions:

1. Cook bacon in a skillet until crispy, then set aside.

2. In the same skillet, scramble the eggs.

3. Assemble the bowl with scrambled eggs, bacon, avocado, cheese, salsa, and season with salt and pepper.

Meal Prep: Can be made fresh in the morning within 20 minutes.

Time: 20 minutes

Nutritional Information:

- Calories: 320

- Protein: 18g

- Fat: 24g

- Carbohydrates: 6g

- Fiber: 3g

Recipe 9: Keto Cinnamon Coconut Flour Porridge

Ingredients:

- 2 tbsp coconut flour

- 1 cup unsweetened coconut milk

- 1/2 tsp cinnamon

- 1 tbsp unsweetened shredded coconut

- 1 tsp vanilla extract

- Low-carb sweetener to taste

Instructions:

1. In a saucepan, heat coconut milk over medium heat.

2. Whisk in coconut flour, cinnamon, shredded coconut, and vanilla extract.

3. Cook, stirring continuously until thickened.

4. Sweeten to taste and serve warm.

Meal Prep: Can be made fresh within 10 minutes.

Time: 10 minutes

Nutritional Information:

- Calories: 180

- Protein: 4g

- Fat: 14g

- Carbohydrates: 8g

- Fiber: 6g

Recipe 10: Keto Turkey Sausage and Egg Casserole

Ingredients:

- 8 oz ground turkey sausage

- 6 eggs

- 1/2 cup heavy cream

- 1 cup spinach

- 1/2 cup shredded cheese

- Salt and pepper to taste

Instructions:

1. Preheat oven to 350°F (175°C).

2. Cook ground turkey sausage in a skillet until browned.

3. Whisk eggs and heavy cream in a bowl, then add spinach, cheese, salt, and pepper.

4. Stir in cooked sausage.

5. Pour the mixture into a greased baking dish.

6. Bake for 25-30 minutes until the center is set.

Meal Prep: Ideal for making ahead and reheating for busy mornings.

Time: 35 minutes

Nutritional Information:

- Calories: 280

- Protein: 18g

- Fat: 20g

- Carbohydrates: 4g

- Fiber: 1g

Recipe 11: Keto Almond Flour Waffles

Ingredients:

- 1 1/2 cups almond flour

- 4 eggs

- 1/4 cup unsweetened almond milk

- 2 tbsp melted butter

- 1 tsp baking powder

- 1/2 tsp vanilla extract

- Low-carb sweetener to taste

Instructions:

1. Preheat waffle iron and grease if necessary.

2. In a bowl, whisk together almond flour, eggs, almond milk, melted butter, baking powder, vanilla extract, and sweetener.

3. Pour the batter into the waffle iron and cook as per the iron's instructions.

Meal Prep: Make a batch, freeze, and reheat in the toaster.

Time: 15 minutes

Nutritional Information:

- Calories: 220

- Protein: 10g

- Fat: 18g

- Carbohydrates: 6g

- Fiber: 3g

Recipe 12: Keto Breakfast Stuffed Peppers

Ingredients:

- 2 bell peppers

- 4 eggs

- 1/2 cup cooked ground sausage

- 1/4 cup diced tomatoes

- 1/4 cup shredded cheese

- Salt and pepper to taste

Instructions:

1. Preheat oven to 375°F (190°C).

2. Cut the tops off the peppers and remove seeds and membranes.

3. In a bowl, mix eggs, sausage, tomatoes, cheese, salt, and pepper.

4. Fill each pepper with the mixture.

5. Bake for 25-30 minutes until the peppers are tender and the filling is set.

Meal Prep: Can be made in advance and reheated for a quick breakfast.

Time: 40 minutes

Nutritional Information:

- Calories: 260

- Protein: 16g

- Fat: 18g

- Carbohydrates: 8g

- Fiber: 2g

Recipe 13: Keto Spinach and Feta Omelette

Ingredients:

- 3 eggs

- 1 cup fresh spinach

- 2 tbsp crumbled feta cheese

- 1 tbsp olive oil

- Salt and pepper to taste

Instructions:

1. Heat olive oil in a skillet over medium heat.

2. Whisk eggs and pour into the skillet.

3. Add spinach, feta, salt, and pepper.

4. Once the bottom is set, fold the omelette in half.

5. Cook for another minute and serve.

Meal Prep: Prepare within 15 minutes for a hearty breakfast.

Time: 15 minutes

Nutritional Information:

- Calories: 240
- Protein: 15g
- Fat: 18g
- Carbohydrates: 4g
- Fiber: 1g

Recipe 14: Keto Peanut Butter Chia Seed Pudding

Ingredients:

- 1/4 cup chia seeds
- 1 cup unsweetened almond milk
- 2 tbsp peanut butter
- 1 tsp cocoa powder (optional)
- Low-carb sweetener to taste

Instructions:

1. Mix chia seeds, almond milk, peanut butter, cocoa powder, and sweetener in a bowl.

2. Stir well and let it sit for 10 minutes.

3. Stir again to prevent clumping.

4. Cover and refrigerate overnight or for at least 4 hours.

5. Serve topped with more peanut butter if desired.

Meal Prep: Prepare the night before for a satisfying morning meal.

Time: 5 minutes (plus overnight refrigeration)

Nutritional Information:

- Calories: 280

- Protein: 10g

- Fat: 20g

- Carbohydrates: 12g

- Fiber: 10g

Recipe 15: Keto Broccoli and Cheese Frittata

Ingredients:

- 6 eggs

- 1 cup chopped broccoli

- 1/2 cup shredded cheese

- 1/4 cup heavy cream

- Salt and pepper to taste

Instructions:

1. Preheat oven to 350°F (175°C).

2. Whisk eggs, heavy cream, salt, and pepper in a bowl.

3. Grease a baking dish and spread broccoli on the bottom.

4. Pour egg mixture over the broccoli.

5. Top with shredded cheese.

6. Bake for 25-30 minutes until the center is set.

Meal Prep: Make ahead and refrigerate for a convenient breakfast.

Time: 35 minutes

Nutritional Information:

- Calories: 280

- Protein: 16g

- Fat: 20g

- Carbohydrates: 6g

- Fiber:

LUNCH RECIPES

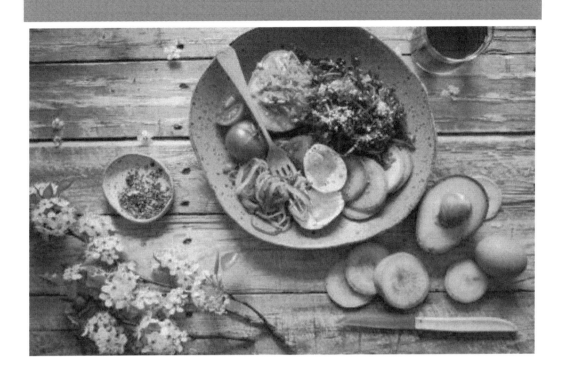

Recipe 1: Grilled Chicken Salad

Ingredients:

- 2 boneless, skinless chicken breasts

- 4 cups mixed salad greens

- 1 cup cherry tomatoes, halved

- 1/2 avocado, sliced

- 2 tablespoons olive oil

- Salt and pepper to taste

Instructions:

1. Preheat grill to medium-high heat.

2. Season chicken breasts with salt and pepper, then grill for

6-8 minutes per side until fully cooked.

3. Let the chicken rest for 5 minutes, then slice into strips.

4. In a large bowl, combine the salad greens, cherry tomatoes, and avocado.

5. Top the salad with grilled chicken strips.

6. Drizzle olive oil over the salad and toss gently to combine.

7. Season with additional salt and pepper if desired.

Meal Prep: Grill chicken ahead of time and store in an airtight container. Assemble the salad just before serving.

Time: 20 minutes

Nutritional Information: Calories: 320 | Fat: 18g | Protein: 30g | Carbs: 9g | Fiber: 5g

Recipe 2: Zucchini Noodles with Pesto

Ingredients:

- 2 medium zucchinis, spiralized

- 1/4 cup pesto sauce

- 1/4 cup grated Parmesan cheese

- 2 tablespoons pine nuts (optional)

Instructions:

1. Heat a skillet over medium heat and add the spiralized zucchini.

2. Sauté for 2-3 minutes until zucchini is tender.

3. Remove from heat and toss with pesto sauce.

4. Sprinkle with Parmesan cheese and pine nuts if desired.

Meal Prep: Spiralize zucchini in advance and store in the refrigerator.

Prepare pesto ahead and keep it refrigerated.

Time: 15 minutes

Nutritional Information: Calories: 210 | Fat: 16g | Protein: 7g | Carbs: 8g | Fiber: 3g

Recipe 3: Tuna Lettuce Wraps

Ingredients:

- 2 cans tuna, drained

- 1/4 cup mayonnaise

- 1/4 cup diced celery

- 1 teaspoon Dijon mustard

- 1 tablespoon lemon juice

- Lettuce leaves for wrapping

Instructions:

1. In a bowl, mix together tuna, mayonnaise, celery, Dijon mustard, and lemon juice.

2. Place a scoop of the tuna mixture onto each lettuce leaf.

3. Roll the lettuce around the filling to create wraps.

Meal Prep: Mix the tuna salad in advance and store in the refrigerator. Assemble the wraps just before eating to prevent the lettuce from wilting.

Time: 10 minutes

Nutritional Information: Calories: 180 | Fat: 10g | Protein: 20g | Carbs: 2g | Fiber: 1g

Recipe 4: Egg Salad Stuffed Bell Peppers

Ingredients:

- 4 hard-boiled eggs, chopped

- 1/4 cup mayonnaise

- 1 tablespoon Dijon mustard

- 2 bell peppers, halved and seeded

- Salt and pepper to taste

Instructions:

1. In a bowl, mix chopped eggs, mayonnaise, and Dijon mustard. Season with salt and pepper.

2. Fill each bell pepper half with the egg salad mixture.

Meal Prep: Prepare the egg salad in advance and store in the refrigerator. Stuff the peppers just before serving.

Time: 15 minutes

Nutritional Information: Calories: 160 | Fat: 12g | Protein: 8g | Carbs: 5g | Fiber: 2g

Recipe 5: Cauliflower Fried Rice

Ingredients:

- 4 cups riced cauliflower

- 1 cup cooked, diced chicken

- 1/2 cup mixed vegetables (peas, carrots, onions)

- 2 eggs, beaten

- 2 tablespoons soy sauce

- 1 tablespoon sesame oil

- Green onions for garnish (optional)

Instructions:

1. In a large skillet, heat sesame oil over medium heat.

2. Add mixed vegetables and sauté until tender.

3. Push vegetables to one side of the skillet, pour beaten eggs on the other side, and scramble.

4. Mix in riced cauliflower and diced chicken, stirring well.

5. Pour soy sauce over the mixture and stir until heated through.

6. Garnish with green onions if desired.

Meal Prep: Prepare riced cauliflower and cooked chicken in advance. Store separately and combine when ready to cook.

Time: 20 minutes

Nutritional Information: Calories: 250 | Fat: 12g | Protein: 20g | Carbs: 10g | Fiber: 5g

Recipe 6: Avocado and Shrimp Salad

Ingredients:

- 1 lb cooked shrimp, peeled and deveined

- 2 avocados, diced

- 1/4 cup red onion, finely chopped

- 2 tablespoons chopped cilantro

- 2 tablespoons olive oil

- 1 tablespoon lime juice

- Salt and pepper to taste

Instructions:

1. In a large bowl, combine shrimp, diced avocados, red onion, and cilantro.

2. Drizzle olive oil and lime juice over the mixture.

3. Season with salt and pepper, then gently toss to combine.

Meal Prep: Cook shrimp in advance and store in the refrigerator. Assemble the salad just before serving.

Time: 15 minutes

Nutritional Information: Calories: 280 | Fat: 18g | Protein: 25g | Carbs: 10g | Fiber: 7g

Recipe 7: Turkey and Cheese Roll-Ups

Ingredients:

- 8 slices turkey breast

- 4 slices cheese (cheddar, Swiss, or any preferred)

- 1/4 cup baby spinach leaves

Instructions:

1. Place two slices of turkey slightly overlapping on a clean surface.

2. Lay a slice of cheese and a few spinach leaves on top of the turkey slices.

3. Roll the turkey and fillings tightly to form a roll-up.

4. Secure with a toothpick if needed.

Meal Prep: Prepare roll-ups in advance and store in an airtight container in the refrigerator.

Time: 5 minutes

Nutritional Information: Calories: 200 | Fat: 12g | Protein: 20g | Carbs: 2g | Fiber: 1g

Recipe 8: Chicken and Broccoli Stir-Fry

Ingredients:

- 2 boneless, skinless chicken thighs, sliced

- 2 cups broccoli florets

- 2 cloves garlic, minced

- 2 tablespoons soy sauce

- 1 tablespoon olive oil

- Sesame seeds for garnish (optional)

Instructions:

1. Heat olive oil in a skillet over medium-high heat.

2. Add chicken slices and cook until browned.

3. Stir in broccoli and minced garlic, sauté until tender.

4. Pour soy sauce over the mixture and cook for an additional minute.

5. Garnish with sesame seeds if desired.

Meal Prep: Slice chicken and chop broccoli in advance. Store separately and combine when ready to cook.

Time: 15 minutes

Nutritional Information: Calories: 280 | Fat: 14g | Protein: 25g | Carbs: 8g | Fiber: 3g

Recipe 9: Salmon Cucumber Rolls

Ingredients:

- 8 oz smoked salmon

- 1 cucumber, peeled into thin strips

- 4 oz cream cheese

- Dill for garnish

Instructions:

1. Lay out strips of cucumber and pat them dry with a paper towel.

2. Spread a thin layer of cream cheese over each strip of cucumber.

3. Place a piece of smoked salmon on each strip and roll up.

4. Secure with a toothpick and garnish with dill.

Meal Prep: Prepare rolls in advance and keep refrigerated until ready to serve.

Time: 10 minutes

Nutritional Information: Calories: 230 | Fat: 15g | Protein: 20g | Carbs: 4g | Fiber: 1g

Recipe 10: Keto Cobb Salad

Ingredients:

- 4 cups mixed salad greens

- 4 slices bacon, cooked and crumbled

- 2 hard-boiled eggs, sliced

- 1/2 cup diced cooked chicken

- 1/4 cup crumbled blue cheese

- 1/4 cup diced avocado

- Ranch dressing (sugar-free)

Instructions:

1. Arrange salad greens in a bowl or on a plate.

2. Top with bacon, sliced eggs, diced chicken, blue cheese, and avocado.

3. Drizzle with ranch dressing.

Meal Prep: Cook bacon, boil eggs, and dice chicken in advance. Assemble the salad just before serving.

Time: 10 minutes

Nutritional Information: Calories: 350 | Fat: 25g | Protein: 22g | Carbs: 6g | Fiber: 3g

Recipe 11: Caprese Stuffed Avocado

Ingredients:

- 2 avocados, halved and pitted

- 1 cup cherry tomatoes, halved

- 4 oz fresh mozzarella, diced

- Fresh basil leaves, chopped

- Balsamic glaze for drizzling

Instructions:

1. Scoop out some avocado from each half to create a larger indentation.

2. In a bowl, mix cherry tomatoes, fresh mozzarella, and chopped basil.

3. Stuff the avocado halves with the Caprese mixture.

4. Drizzle with balsamic glaze before serving.

Meal Prep: Prepare Caprese mixture in advance and refrigerate. Fill avocados just before serving.

Time: 10 minutes

Nutritional Information: Calories: 280 | Fat: 22g | Protein: 10g | Carbs: 12g | Fiber: 8g

Recipe 12: Chicken Lettuce Cups

Ingredients:

- 1 lb ground chicken

- 1/4 cup chopped water chestnuts

- 2 tablespoons soy sauce

- 1 tablespoon sesame oil

- Butter lettuce leaves for wrapping

Instructions:

1. In a skillet over medium heat, cook ground chicken until browned.

2. Add water chestnuts, soy sauce, and sesame oil, stirring well.

3. Spoon the chicken mixture into lettuce leaves for wrapping.

Meal Prep: Cook chicken mixture in advance and store in the refrigerator. Assemble lettuce cups just before serving.

Time: 15 minutes

Nutritional Information: Calories: 260 | Fat: 15g | Protein: 25g | Carbs: 5g | Fiber: 1g

Recipe 13: Spinach and Feta Stuffed Mushrooms

Ingredients:

- 12 large mushrooms, stems removed

- 1 cup fresh spinach, chopped

- 1/2 cup crumbled feta cheese

- 2 cloves garlic, minced

- 2 tablespoons olive oil

Instructions:

1. Preheat the oven to 375°F (190°C).

2. In a bowl, mix together chopped spinach, feta cheese, minced garlic, and olive oil.

3. Stuff each mushroom cap with the spinach and feta mixture.

4. Place stuffed mushrooms on a baking sheet and bake for 15-18 minutes.

Meal Prep: Prepare the filling in advance and refrigerate. Fill mushrooms and bake when ready to serve.

Time: 25 minutes

Nutritional Information: Calories: 180 | Fat: 14g | Protein: 6g | Carbs: 8g | Fiber: 2g

Recipe 14: Beef Lettuce Wraps

Ingredients:

- 1 lb ground beef

- 1/4 cup chopped bell peppers

- 2 tablespoons coconut aminos (or soy sauce)

- 1 tablespoon sesame oil

- Iceberg lettuce leaves for wrapping

Instructions:

1. In a skillet over medium heat, brown the ground beef.

2. Add chopped bell peppers, coconut aminos, and sesame oil, stirring well.

3. Spoon the beef mixture into lettuce leaves for wrapping.

Meal Prep: Cook beef mixture in advance and store in the refrigerator. Assemble lettuce wraps just before serving.

Time: 15 minutes

Nutritional Information: Calories: 290 | Fat: 20g | Protein: 22g | Carbs: 4g | Fiber: 1g

Recipe 15: Tofu Stir-Fry

Ingredients:

- 1 block firm tofu, diced

- 2 cups mixed vegetables (broccoli, bell peppers, snap peas)

- 2 tablespoons soy sauce

- 1 tablespoon sesame oil

- 1 teaspoon ginger, grated

Instructions:

1. Heat sesame oil in a skillet over medium heat.

2. Add diced tofu and cook until lightly browned on all sides.

3. Stir in mixed vegetables and grated ginger, sauté until tender.

4. Pour soy sauce over the mixture and cook for an additional minute.

Meal Prep: Dice tofu and chop vegetables in advance. Store separately and combine when ready to cook.

Time: 20 minutes

Nutritional Information: Calories: 240 | Fat: 14g | Protein: 18g | Carbs: 10g | Fiber: 4g

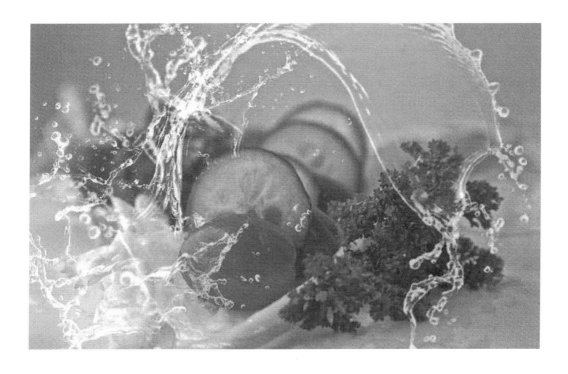

DINNER RECIPES

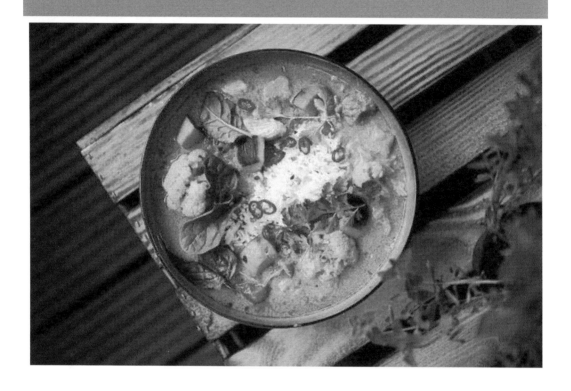

Recipe 1: Lemon Garlic Butter Salmon

Ingredients:

- 4 salmon fillets

- 4 tablespoons butter

- 4 cloves garlic, minced

- 2 tablespoons lemon juice

- Salt and pepper to taste

- Fresh parsley, chopped for garnish

Instructions:

1. Preheat the oven to 375°F.

2. Place salmon fillets on a baking sheet lined with parchment paper.

3. In a saucepan, melt butter and add minced garlic. Cook until fragrant.

4. Stir in lemon juice, salt, and pepper. Pour the mixture over the salmon.

5. Bake for 12-15 minutes or until the salmon easily flakes with a fork.

6. Garnish with fresh parsley and serve.

Meal Prep: Ready in 25 minutes. Serve with roasted vegetables for a complete meal.

Time: 25 minutes

Nutritional Information:

- Calories: 320

- Fat: 20g

- Protein: 34g

- Carbohydrates: 2g

Recipe 2: Zucchini Noodles with Pesto

Ingredients:

- 4 medium zucchinis, spiralized

- 1/2 cup basil pesto

- 1 tablespoon olive oil

- 1/4 cup pine nuts

- Grated Parmesan cheese (optional)

- Salt and pepper to taste

Instructions:

1. Heat olive oil in a pan over medium heat.

2. Add zucchini noodles and cook for 2-3 minutes until tender.

3. Toss in basil pesto and pine nuts. Stir until combined.

4. Season with salt and pepper.

5. Optional: Sprinkle with grated Parmesan cheese before serving.

Meal Prep: Quick and easy, serve as a main or a side dish.

Time: 15 minutes

Nutritional Information:

- Calories: 180
- Fat: 15g
- Protein: 5g
- Carbohydrates: 8g

Recipe 3: Grilled Lemon Herb Chicken

Ingredients:

- 4 chicken breasts
- 2 tablespoons olive oil
- 2 tablespoons fresh lemon juice
- 2 cloves garlic, minced
- 1 teaspoon dried thyme
- 1 teaspoon dried rosemary
- Salt and pepper to taste

Instructions:

1. Preheat grill to medium-high heat.
2. In a bowl, mix olive oil, lemon juice, minced garlic, thyme, and rosemary.
3. Season chicken breasts with salt and pepper, then coat with the marinade.
4. Grill the chicken for 6-8 minutes per side until cooked through.
5. Remove from grill and let it rest for a few minutes before serving.

Meal Prep: Great for meal prepping; serve with a side salad or roasted vegetables.

Time: 30 minutes

Nutritional Information:

- Calories: 250

- Fat: 10g

- Protein: 35g

- Carbohydrates: 2g

Recipe 4: Cauliflower Crust Pizza

Ingredients:

- 1 head cauliflower, grated or processed into "rice"

- 1 cup mozzarella cheese, shredded

- 1 egg

- 1 teaspoon dried oregano

- 1/2 teaspoon garlic powder

- Tomato sauce, cheese, and toppings of choice

Instructions:

1. Preheat oven to 400°F.

2. Steam or microwave cauliflower rice, then let it cool.

3. Mix cauliflower, mozzarella, egg, oregano, and garlic powder in a bowl to form a dough.

4. Press the dough onto a baking sheet lined with parchment paper to create a crust.

5. Bake for 15-20 minutes until the crust is golden.

6. Add tomato sauce, cheese, and desired toppings. Bake until cheese melts.

Meal Prep: Ideal for a family dinner or meal prepping for the week.

Time: 40 minutes

Nutritional Information:

- Calories: 220 (per slice, excluding toppings)

- Fat: 14g

- Protein: 18g

- Carbohydrates: 8g

Recipe 5: Spinach and Feta Stuffed Chicken

Ingredients:

- 4 chicken breasts

- 1 cup spinach, chopped

- 1/2 cup feta cheese

- 2 cloves garlic, minced

- Salt and pepper to taste

- Olive oil for cooking

Instructions:

1. Preheat oven to 375°F.

2. Cut a pocket into each chicken breast without cutting all the way through.

3. In a bowl, mix spinach, feta, garlic, salt, and pepper.

4. Stuff each chicken breast with the spinach and feta mixture.

5. Heat oil in a pan and sear both sides of the chicken for 2-3 minutes.

6. Transfer chicken to a baking dish and bake for 20-25 minutes until cooked through.

Meal Prep: Serve with a side of roasted vegetables or a fresh salad.

Time: 35 minutes

Nutritional Information:

- Calories: 280

- Fat: 12g

- Protein: 36g

- Carbohydrates: 4g

Recipe 6: Beef and Broccoli Stir-Fry

Ingredients:

- 1 lb beef sirloin, thinly sliced

- 2 cups broccoli florets

- 3 tablespoons soy sauce

- 2 tablespoons sesame oil

- 2 cloves garlic, minced

- 1 teaspoon ginger, grated

- Sesame seeds for garnish

Instructions:

1. In a bowl, marinate beef in soy sauce, sesame oil, garlic, and ginger for 15 minutes.

2. Heat a pan over medium-high heat and add marinated beef. Cook until browned.

3. Add broccoli to the pan and stir-fry for 3-4 minutes.

4. Serve the beef and broccoli over cauliflower rice or on its own.

5. Garnish with sesame seeds.

Meal Prep: Serve hot as a main dish or use it as a meal prep option for a few days.

Time: 20 minutes

Nutritional Information:

- Calories: 310

- Fat: 20g

- Protein: 30g

- Carbohydrates: 6g

Recipe 7: Creamy Tuscan Shrimp

Ingredients:

- 1 lb shrimp, peeled and deveined

- 2 tablespoons butter

- 4 cloves garlic, minced

- 1 cup heavy cream

- 1/2 cup grated Parmesan cheese

- 1 cup sun-dried tomatoes

- Fresh basil for garnish

- Salt and pepper to taste

Instructions:

1. In a pan, melt butter and sauté garlic until fragrant.

2. Add shrimp and cook until pink, then set aside.

3. In the same pan, pour in heavy cream and let it simmer.

4. Add Parmesan cheese and sun-dried tomatoes, stir until thickened.

5. Return shrimp to the pan, mix, and cook for 2 minutes.

6. Garnish with fresh basil before serving.

Meal Prep: Enjoy with zoodles or a side of steamed vegetables.

Time: 25 minutes

Nutritional Information:

- Calories: 340

- Fat: 25g

- Protein: 25g

- Carbohydrates: 8g

Recipe 8: Avocado and Bacon Stuffed Burgers

Ingredients:

- 1 lb ground beef

- 4 slices bacon, cooked and crumbled

- 2 avocados, mashed

- 1/2 teaspoon garlic powder

- Salt and pepper to taste

- Lettuce leaves for wrapping

Instructions:

1. In a bowl, mix ground beef, bacon, garlic powder, salt, and pepper.

2. Form the mixture into burger patties.

3. Make an indentation in the center of each patty and fill with mashed avocado.

4. Grill the burgers for 4-5 minutes per side until cooked through.

5. Serve in lettuce leaves instead of buns.

Meal Prep: Serve with a side salad or roasted veggies.

Time: 30 minutes

Nutritional Information:

- Calories: 380

- Fat: 25g

- Protein: 30g

- Carbohydrates: 6g

Recipe 9: Eggplant Lasagna

Ingredients:

- 2 large eggplants, sliced lengthwise

- 1 lb ground turkey

- 2 cups marinara sauce

- 1 cup ricotta cheese

- 1 cup mozzarella cheese, shredded

- 1/4 cup grated Parmesan cheese

- Italian seasoning, salt, and pepper

Instructions:

1. Preheat oven to 375°F.

2. Roast eggplant slices in the oven for 15 minutes.

3. In a pan, brown ground turkey and season with Italian seasoning, salt, and pepper.

4. In a baking dish, layer marinara sauce, roasted eggplant, turkey, ricotta, and mozzarella.

5. Repeat the layers and finish with a layer of mozzarella and Parmesan on top.

6. Bake for 25-30 minutes until cheese is golden and bubbly.

Meal Prep: Ideal for dinner and leftovers for lunch.

Time: 50 minutes

Nutritional Information:

- Calories: 320

- Fat: 18g

- Protein: 25g

- Carbohydrates: 14g

Recipe 10: Lemon Garlic Butter Shrimp

Ingredients:

- 1 lb shrimp, peeled and deveined

- 4 tablespoons butter

- 4 cloves garlic, minced

- 2 tablespoons lemon juice

- Fresh parsley for garnish

- Salt and pepper to taste

Instructions:

1. In a pan, melt butter and add minced garlic. Cook until fragrant.

2. Add shrimp and sauté for 2-3 minutes until pink and opaque.

3. Stir in lemon juice, salt, and pepper.

4. Garnish with fresh parsley before serving.

Meal Prep: Serve with cauliflower rice or a side of mixed greens.

Time: 15 minutes

Nutritional Information:

- Calories: 220

- Fat: 15g

- Protein: 20g

- Carbohydrates: 2g

Recipe 11: Pork Tenderloin with Dijon Sauce

Ingredients:

- 1 lb pork tenderloin

- 2 tablespoons Dijon mustard

- 2 tablespoons olive oil

- 2 cloves garlic, minced

- 1/4 cup chicken broth

- Fresh thyme for garnish

- Salt and pepper to taste

Instructions:

1. Preheat oven to 400°F.

2. Season pork with salt and pepper.

3. In an oven-safe skillet, heat olive oil over medium-high heat.

4. Sear the pork on all sides until golden brown.

5. Transfer skillet to the oven and roast for 15-20 minutes.

6. Remove pork and let it rest. In the same skillet, sauté garlic, then add Dijon and broth. Simmer until thickened.

7. Slice the pork and serve with Dijon sauce. Garnish with fresh thyme.

Meal Prep: Pair with steamed vegetables for a balanced meal.

Time: 35 minutes

Nutritional Information:

- Calories: 280

- Fat: 15g

- Protein: 30g

- Carbohydrates: 2g

Recipe 12: Cabbage and Sausage Skillet

Ingredients:

- 1 lb sausage, sliced

- 1 small head cabbage, shredded

- 1 onion, chopped

- 2 cloves garlic, minced

- 1 teaspoon paprika

- Salt and pepper to taste

Instructions:

1. In a skillet, brown sausage over medium heat, then set aside.

2. In the same skillet, sauté onions and garlic until soft.

3. Add shredded cabbage and cook until tender.

4. Stir in paprika, salt, and pepper. Add the cooked sausage back to the skillet.

5. Mix everything well and cook for a few more minutes.

Meal Prep: Serve hot or pack for lunch the next day.

Time: 30 minutes

Nutritional Information:

- Calories: 320

- Fat: 25g

- Protein: 15g

- Carbohydrates: 10g

Recipe 13: Stuffed Bell Peppers

Ingredients:

- 4 bell peppers

- 1 lb ground beef

- 1 cup cauliflower rice

- 1 cup marinara sauce

- 1/2 cup shredded mozzarella

- Italian seasoning, salt, and pepper

Instructions:

1. Preheat oven to 375°F.

2. Cut the tops off the bell peppers and remove seeds and membranes.

3. In a pan, brown ground beef, then mix in cauliflower rice and marinara sauce.

4. Season the beef mixture with Italian seasoning, salt, and pepper.

5. Stuff the bell peppers with the mixture and place in a baking dish.

6. Top each pepper with shredded mozzarella and bake for 25-30 minutes.

Meal Prep: Enjoy as a complete meal or pair with a fresh salad.

Time: 45 minutes

Nutritional Information:

- Calories: 290

- Fat: 18g

- Protein: 20g

- Carbohydrates: 10g

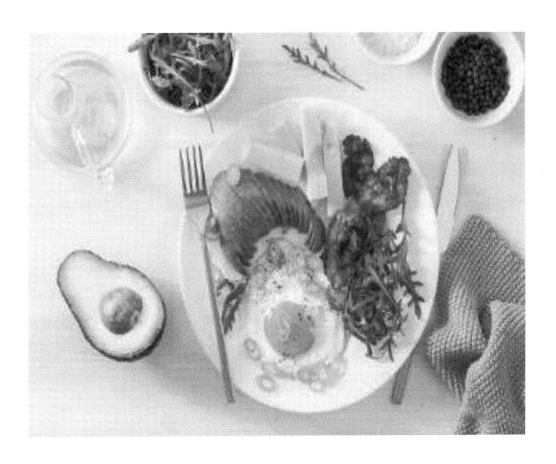

SIDE DISHES

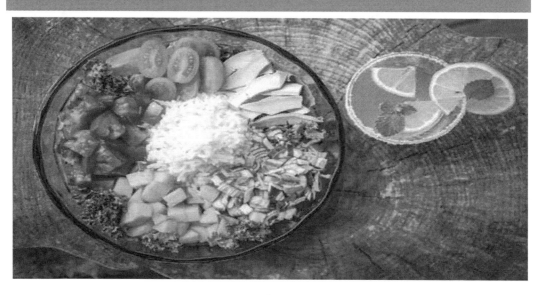

1. Garlic Parmesan Roasted Broccoli

Ingredients:

- 1 head of broccoli, cut into florets

- 2 tablespoons olive oil

- 2 cloves garlic, minced

- 1/4 cup grated Parmesan cheese

- Salt and pepper to taste

Instruction:

1. Preheat the oven to 400°F (200°C).

2. Toss broccoli florets with olive oil, garlic, salt, and pepper.

3. Spread the broccoli on a baking sheet and roast for 20-25 minutes.

4. Sprinkle Parmesan cheese over the broccoli and roast for an additional 5 minutes.

Meal Prep: Ready in 30-35 minutes.

Nutritional Info: Calories: 120 | Net Carbs: 4g | Protein: 6g | Fat: 9g

2. Zucchini Noodles with Pesto

Ingredients:

- 2 medium zucchinis, spiralized
- 1/2 cup basil pesto
- 1/4 cup cherry tomatoes, halved
- 2 tablespoons pine nuts (optional)
- Salt and pepper to taste

Instruction:

1. Spiralize the zucchinis into noodles and set aside.
2. In a pan, heat the pesto and add zucchini noodles, tossing to coat.
3. Cook for 3-5 minutes until the noodles are tender.

4. Garnish with cherry tomatoes, pine nuts, salt, and pepper.

Meal Prep: Ready in 15 minutes.

Nutritional Info: Calories: 180 | Net Carbs: 6g | Protein: 4g | Fat: 15g

3. Cauliflower "Mac" and Cheese

Ingredients:

- 1 head cauliflower, cut into florets
- 1 cup heavy cream
- 1 1/2 cups shredded cheddar cheese
- 1/4 cup grated Parmesan cheese
- 1/4 teaspoon mustard powder
- Salt and pepper to taste

Instruction:

1. Steam or boil cauliflower until tender, then drain and set aside.

2. In a saucepan, heat heavy cream and stir in cheddar and Parmesan cheese until melted.

3. Add mustard powder, salt, and pepper, then mix in the cauliflower.

4. Bake at 350°F (175°C) for 15-20 minutes until bubbly.

Meal Prep: Ready in 40-45 minutes.
Nutritional Info: Calories: 280 | Net Carbs: 8g | Protein: 12g | Fat: 22g

4. Avocado Cucumber Salad

Ingredients:

- 2 avocados, diced

- 2 cucumbers, sliced

- 1/4 cup red onion, thinly sliced

- 2 tablespoons olive oil

- 1 tablespoon lemon juice

- Fresh dill, chopped

- Salt and pepper to taste

Instruction:

1. In a bowl, combine avocados, cucumbers, and red onion.

2. In a separate bowl, mix olive oil, lemon juice, dill, salt, and pepper.

3. Drizzle the dressing over the salad and gently toss to combine.

Meal Prep: Ready in 10 minutes.
Nutritional Info: Calories: 160 | Net Carbs: 8g | Protein: 2g | Fat: 14g

5. Mushroom Cauliflower Risotto

Ingredients:

- 1 head cauliflower, riced

- 2 cups mushrooms, sliced

- 2 cloves garlic, minced

- 1/2 cup chicken or vegetable broth

- 1/4 cup heavy cream

- 1/4 cup grated Parmesan cheese

- Fresh thyme, chopped

- Salt and pepper to taste

Instruction:

1. In a pan, sauté mushrooms and garlic until tender.

2. Add riced cauliflower, broth, and simmer until the cauliflower is cooked.

3. Stir in heavy cream, Parmesan, thyme, salt, and pepper.

4. Cook for an additional 5 minutes until creamy.

Meal Prep: Ready in 25 minutes.
Nutritional Info: Calories: 210 | Net Carbs: 6g | Protein: 9g | Fat: 16g

6. Crispy Baked Asparagus Fries

Ingredients:

- 1 bunch asparagus, trimmed

- 1/2 cup almond flour

- 1/4 cup grated Parmesan cheese

- 2 eggs, beaten

- 1 teaspoon garlic powder

- Salt and pepper to taste

Instruction:

1. Preheat the oven to 425°F (220°C) and line a baking sheet with parchment paper.

2. Mix almond flour, Parmesan, garlic powder, salt, and pepper in one bowl.

3. Dip asparagus in beaten eggs, then coat with the almond flour mixture.

4. Place the asparagus on the baking sheet and bake for 12-15 minutes until crispy.

Meal Prep: Ready in 20 minutes.
Nutritional Info: Calories: 140 | Net Carbs: 5g | Protein: 8g | Fat: 9g

7. Cabbage and Bacon Saute

Ingredients:

- 4 cups cabbage, shredded
- 4 slices bacon, chopped
- 1 onion, sliced
- 2 cloves garlic, minced
- 2 tablespoons apple cider vinegar
- Salt and pepper to taste

Instruction:

1. In a pan, cook bacon until crispy, then remove and set aside.

2. Sauté onion and garlic in the bacon grease until softened.

3. Add cabbage, apple cider vinegar, salt, and pepper, and cook until cabbage is tender.

4. Stir in the cooked bacon before serving.

Meal Prep: Ready in 20 minutes.
Nutritional Info: Calories: 200 | Net Carbs: 6g | Protein: 7g | Fat: 15g

8. Eggplant Caprese Skewers

Ingredients:

- 1 large eggplant, cut into cubes
- 1 cup cherry tomatoes
- 8 ounces fresh mozzarella, cut into cubes
- Fresh basil leaves
- Balsamic glaze (optional)
- Salt and pepper to taste

Instruction:

1. Season eggplant cubes with salt and pepper, then grill or roast until tender.

2. Assemble skewers by threading eggplant, cherry tomatoes, mozzarella, and basil leaves.

3. Drizzle with balsamic glaze if desired before serving.

Meal Prep: Ready in 25 minutes.
Nutritional Info: Calories: 170 | Net Carbs: 6g | Protein: 9g | Fat: 12g

9. Brussels Sprouts with Bacon and Balsamic

Ingredients:

- 4 cups Brussels sprouts, halved

- 4 slices bacon, chopped

- 2 tablespoons balsamic vinegar

- 2 tablespoons olive oil

- Salt and pepper to taste

Instruction:

1. In a pan, cook bacon until crispy, then remove and set aside.

2. Sauté Brussels sprouts in bacon fat and olive oil until slightly caramelized.

3. Drizzle with balsamic vinegar, add cooked bacon, and toss to coat.

Meal Prep: Ready in 20 minutes.
Nutritional Info: Calories: 190 | Net Carbs: 8g | Protein: 7g | Fat: 14g

10. Spinach and Feta Stuffed Mushrooms

Ingredients:

- 12 large mushrooms, stems removed

- 2 cups spinach, chopped

- 1/2 cup feta cheese, crumbled

- 2 cloves garlic, minced

- 2 tablespoons olive oil

- Salt and pepper to taste

Instruction:

1. Preheat the oven to 375°F (190°C) and line a baking sheet with parchment paper.

2. Sauté spinach and garlic in olive oil until wilted.

3. Mix the cooked spinach with feta, salt, and pepper, then stuff into mushroom caps.

4. Bake for 15-20 minutes until mushrooms are tender.

Meal Prep: Ready in 25 minutes. **Nutritional Info:** Calories: 160 | Net Carbs: 5g | Protein: 6g | Fat: 12g

11. Cauliflower Rice Pilaf

Ingredients:

- 1 head cauliflower, riced

- 1/4 cup almonds, chopped

- 1/4 cup dried cranberries (unsweetened)

- 2 tablespoons butter

- 1 teaspoon curry powder

- Salt and pepper to taste

Instruction:

1. In a pan, melt butter and sauté cauliflower rice until slightly golden.

2. Add chopped almonds, dried cranberries, curry powder, salt, and pepper.

3. Cook for 5-7 minutes until flavors meld together.

Meal Prep: Ready in 15 minutes. **Nutritional Info:** Calories: 190 | Net Carbs: 7g | Protein: 5g | Fat: 14g

12. Lemon Garlic Green Beans

Ingredients:

- 1 pound green beans, trimmed

- 2 tablespoons olive oil

- 2 cloves garlic, minced

- Zest of 1 lemon

- Salt and pepper to taste

Instruction:

1. Blanch green beans in boiling water for 2-3 minutes, then transfer to ice water.

2. In a pan, heat olive oil and sauté garlic until fragrant.

3. Add green beans, lemon zest, salt, and pepper, and sauté for 3-5 minutes.

Meal Prep: Ready in 15 minutes.
Nutritional Info: Calories: 120 | Net Carbs: 6g | Protein: 2g | Fat: 10g

13. Cucumber Radish Salad

Ingredients:

- 2 cucumbers, thinly sliced

- 1 cup radishes, thinly sliced

- 1/4 cup sour cream or Greek yogurt

- 2 tablespoons white wine vinegar

- Fresh dill, chopped

- Salt and pepper to taste

Instruction:

1. In a bowl, combine sliced cucumbers and radishes.

2. Mix sour cream or yogurt, white wine vinegar, dill, salt, and pepper for the dressing.

3. Toss the dressing with the vegetables until coated.

Meal Prep: Ready in 10 minutes.
Nutritional Info: Calories: 100 | Net Carbs: 5g | Protein: 2g | Fat: 8g

14. Parmesan Roasted Brussels Sprouts

Ingredients:

- 4 cups Brussels sprouts, halved

- 1/4 cup grated Parmesan cheese

- 2 tablespoons olive oil

- 2 cloves garlic, minced

- Salt and pepper to taste

Instruction:

1. Preheat the oven to 400°F (200°C).

2. Toss Brussels sprouts with olive oil, garlic, salt, and pepper.

3. Spread on a baking sheet and roast for 20-25 minutes.

4. Sprinkle with Parmesan cheese and roast for an additional 5 minutes.

Meal Prep: Ready in 30-35 minutes.
Nutritional Info: Calories: 150 | Net Carbs: 7g | Protein: 6g | Fat: 10g

15. Mashed Cauliflower with Herbs

Ingredients:

- 1 head cauliflower, cut into florets

- 1/4 cup cream cheese

- 2 tablespoons butter

- Fresh herbs (parsley, chives, thyme)

- Salt and pepper to taste

Instruction:

1. Steam or boil cauliflower until tender, then drain well.

2. Blend cauliflower, cream cheese, butter, herbs, salt, and pepper until smooth.

Meal Prep: Ready in 20 minutes.
Nutritional Info: Calories: 160 | Net Carbs: 6g | Protein: 4g | Fat: 12g

16. Eggplant Tomato Bake

Ingredients:

- 2 large eggplants, sliced

- 2 cups sugar-free marinara sauce

- 1 cup mozzarella cheese, shredded

- Fresh basil leaves

- Salt and pepper to taste

Instruction:

1. Preheat the oven to 375°F (190°C).

2. Layer eggplant slices in a baking dish, season with salt and pepper.

3. Spread marinara sauce over the eggplant, top with mozzarella, and repeat the layers.

4. Bake for 30-35 minutes until cheese is bubbly and golden.

5. Garnish with fresh basil before serving.

Meal Prep: Ready in 40-45 minutes.
Nutritional Info: Calories: 220 | Net Carbs: 9g | Protein: 10g | Fat: 15g

17. Kale and Bacon Saute

Ingredients:

- 4 cups kale, chopped

- 4 slices bacon, chopped

- 2 cloves garlic, minced

- 2 tablespoons apple cider vinegar

- Salt and pepper to taste

Instruction:

1. In a pan, cook bacon until crispy, then remove and set aside.

2. Sauté garlic in the bacon grease until fragrant.

3. Add kale, apple cider vinegar, salt, and pepper, and cook until wilted.

4. Stir in the cooked bacon before serving.

Meal Prep: Ready in 15 minutes.
Nutritional Info: Calories: 180 | Net Carbs: 5g | Protein: 8g | Fat: 12g

SNACKS RECIPES

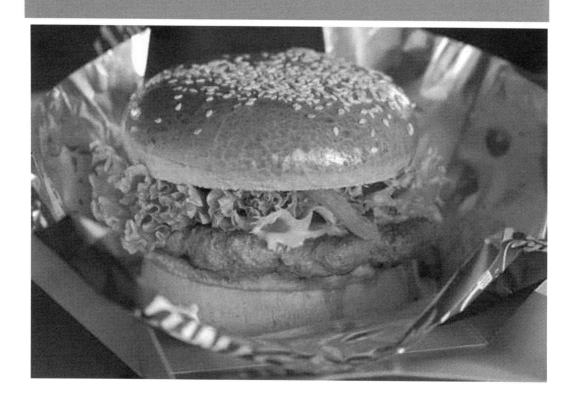

Recipe 1: Keto Pepperoni Chips

Ingredients:

- Pepperoni slices

- Olive oil

Instructions:

1. Preheat the oven to 400°F (200°C).

2. Blot excess oil from the pepperoni slices using a paper towel.

3. Place the pepperoni slices on a baking sheet lined with parchment paper.

4. Lightly brush the slices with olive oil.

~ 63 ~

5. Bake for 8-10 minutes until crispy.

6. Let cool and serve.

Meal Prep: Quick and easy, ideal for immediate consumption.

Time: 15 minutes

Nutritional Information:

- Calories: 120

- Fat: 10g

- Protein: 7g

- Carbs: 1g

Recipe 2: Avocado Stuffed Eggs

Ingredients:

- Hard-boiled eggs

- Ripe avocados

- Lemon juice

- Salt and pepper

- Paprika (optional)

Instructions:

1. Cut hard-boiled eggs in half lengthwise and remove yolks.

2. In a bowl, mash egg yolks with ripe avocado and a splash of lemon juice.

3. Season with salt and pepper.

4. Spoon or pipe the mixture into the egg white halves.

5. Sprinkle with paprika if desired.

Meal Prep: Keep refrigerated for up to 24 hours.

Time: 20 minutes

Nutritional Information:

- Calories: 150

- Fat: 12g

- Protein: 8g

- Carbs: 4g

Recipe 3: Zucchini Parmesan Crisps

Ingredients:

- Zucchini

- Grated Parmesan cheese

- Olive oil

- Garlic powder

- Salt and pepper

Instructions:

1. Preheat the oven to 425°F (220°C).

2. Slice the zucchini into thin rounds.

3. In a bowl, mix zucchini with olive oil, garlic powder, salt, and pepper.

4. Coat zucchini slices with grated Parmesan cheese.

5. Place slices on a baking sheet lined with parchment paper.

6. Bake for 15-20 minutes until golden and crispy.

Meal Prep: Best when consumed immediately.

Time: 25 minutes

Nutritional Information:

- Calories: 90

- Fat: 6g

- Protein: 5g

- Carbs: 3g

Recipe 4: Cauliflower Hummus

Ingredients:

- Cauliflower florets

- Tahini

- Garlic

- Lemon juice

- Olive oil

- Cumin

- Salt

Instructions:

1. Steam or roast cauliflower until tender.

2. Blend cauliflower, tahini, garlic, lemon juice, olive oil, cumin, and salt until smooth.

3. Adjust seasonings as per taste.

Meal Prep: Refrigerate in an airtight container for up to 3 days.

Time: 30 minutes

Nutritional Information:

- Calories: 70

- Fat: 5g

- Protein: 3g

- Carbs: 4g

Recipe 5: Bacon-Wrapped Asparagus

Ingredients:

- Fresh asparagus spears

- Bacon slices

- Olive oil

- Salt and pepper

Instructions:

1. Preheat the oven to 400°F (200°C).

2. Coat asparagus spears in olive oil, salt, and pepper.

3. Wrap a slice of bacon around each asparagus spear.

4. Place on a baking sheet and bake for 20-25 minutes.

Meal Prep: Best when served fresh.

Time: 30 minutes

Nutritional Information:

- Calories: 120

- Fat: 9g

- Protein: 6g

- Carbs: 3g

Recipe 6: Cheese Crisps

Ingredients:

- Shredded cheese (cheddar, parmesan, etc.)

Instructions:

1. Preheat the oven to 375°F (190°C).

2. Line a baking sheet with parchment paper.

3. Place small piles of shredded cheese on the sheet, leaving space between them.

4. Bake for 6-8 minutes until the edges are golden.

5. Let cool to crisp up before serving.

Meal Prep: Store in an airtight container for up to 3 days.

Time: 15 minutes

Nutritional Information:

- Calories: 100

- Fat: 8g

- Protein: 7g

- Carbs: 1g

Recipe 7: Coconut Fat Bombs

Ingredients:

- Coconut oil

- Unsweetened shredded coconut

- Stevia or other keto-friendly sweetener

- Vanilla extract (optional)

Instructions:

1. Melt the coconut oil in a saucepan over low heat.

2. Mix in shredded coconut and sweetener, add vanilla if desired.

3. Pour into molds or an ice cube tray and freeze until set.

Meal Prep: Store in the freezer for up to a month.

Time: 10 minutes

Nutritional Information:

- Calories: 90
- Fat: 9g
- Protein: 0g
- Carbs: 1g

Recipe 8: Cucumber Smoked Salmon Bites

Ingredients:

- English cucumber
- Smoked salmon slices
- Cream cheese
- Fresh dill

Instructions:

1. Slice the cucumber into rounds.
2. Spread a small amount of cream cheese on each cucumber round.
3. Top with a piece of smoked salmon.
4. Garnish with fresh dill.

Meal Prep: Ideal for immediate consumption.

Time: 15 minutes

Nutritional Information:

- Calories: 70
- Fat: 5g
- Protein: 4g
- Carbs: 2g

Recipe 9: Almond Butter Fat Bombs

Ingredients:

- Almond butter
- Coconut oil

- Stevia or other keto-friendly sweetener

Instructions:

1. Mix almond butter, melted coconut oil, and sweetener in a bowl.

2. Pour the mixture into silicone molds or an ice cube tray.

3. Freeze until solid.

Meal Prep: Store in the freezer for up to a month.

Time: 10 minutes

Nutritional Information:

- Calories: 80

- Fat: 7g

- Protein: 2g

- Carbs: 2g

Recipe 10: Kale Chips

Ingredients:

- Fresh kale

- Olive oil

- Salt and pepper

Instructions:

1. Preheat the oven to 275°F (135°C).

2. Remove kale leaves from stems and tear into bite-sized pieces.

3. Toss the kale with olive oil, salt, and pepper.

4. Spread the kale in a single layer on a baking sheet.

5. Bake for 15-20 minutes until crispy.

Meal Prep: Consume immediately for best taste and texture.

Time: 25 minutes

Nutritional Information:

- Calories: 50

- Fat: 3g

- Protein: 2g

- Carbs: 4g

Recipe 11: Prosciutto-Wrapped Mozzarella Sticks

Ingredients:

- Mozzarella sticks

- Prosciutto slices

Instructions:

1. Wrap a slice of prosciutto around each mozzarella stick.

2. Optionally, secure with a toothpick.

3. Heat a skillet over medium heat and cook the wrapped sticks until the prosciutto is crispy.

Meal Prep: Best served fresh.

Time: 10 minutes

Nutritional Information:

- Calories: 110

- Fat: 8g

- Protein: 10g

- Carbs: 1g

Recipe 12: Turmeric Spiced Nuts

Ingredients:

- Mixed nuts (almonds, walnuts, pecans, etc.)

- Turmeric

- Olive oil

- Salt

Instructions:

1. Preheat the oven to 325°F (165°C).

2. In a bowl, toss the nuts with olive oil, turmeric, and salt.

3. Spread the nuts on a baking sheet.

4. Bake for 15-20 minutes, stirring occasionally.

Meal Prep: Store in an airtight container for up to two weeks.

Time: 25 minutes

Nutritional Information:

- Calories: 160

- Fat: 14g

- Protein: 6g

- Carbs: 4g

Recipe 13: Eggplant Chips

Ingredients:

- Eggplant

- Olive oil

- Italian seasoning

- Garlic powder

- Salt and pepper

Instructions:

1. Preheat the oven to 375°F (190°C).

2. Slice the eggplant into thin rounds.

3. Toss slices in olive oil, Italian seasoning, garlic powder, salt, and pepper.

4. Place on a baking sheet and bake for 20-25 minutes until crispy.

Meal Prep: Best when consumed immediately.

Time: 30 minutes

Nutritional Information:

- Calories: 70

- Fat: 5g

- Protein: 2g

- Carbs: 6g

Recipe 14: Spicy Guacamole Deviled Eggs

Ingredients:

- Hard-boiled eggs

- Ripe avocados

- Lime juice

- Red pepper flakes

- Cilantro

- Salt

Instructions:

1. Cut hard-boiled eggs in half lengthwise and remove yolks.

2. In a bowl, mash egg yolks with ripe avocado, lime juice, red pepper flakes, and salt.

3. Spoon or pipe the mixture into the egg white halves.

4. Garnish with cilantro.

Meal Prep: Keep refrigerated for up to 24 hours.

Time: 20 minutes

Nutritional Information:

- Calories: 140

- Fat: 11g

- Protein: 8g

- Carbs: 4g

Recipe 15: Parmesan Crusted Cauliflower

Ingredients:

- Cauliflower florets

- Grated Parmesan cheese

- Almond flour

- Eggs

- Garlic powder

- Salt and pepper

Instructions:

1. Preheat the oven to 425°F (220°C).

2. In one bowl, beat eggs. In another bowl, mix Parmesan, almond flour, garlic powder, salt, and pepper.

3. Dip cauliflower in egg, then coat with the Parmesan mixture.

4. Place on a baking sheet and bake for 20-25 minutes until golden.

Meal Prep: Consume immediately for best taste and texture.

Time: 30 minutes

Nutritional Information:

- Calories: 100

- Fat: 7g

- Protein: 6g

- Carbs: 4g

Recipe 16: Baked Cheese Stuffed Jalapeños

Ingredients:

- Jalapeños

- Cream cheese

- Shredded cheddar cheese

Instructions:

1. Preheat the oven to 375°F (190°C).

2. Cut jalapeños in half lengthwise and remove seeds.

3. Fill each jalapeño half with cream cheese and sprinkle cheddar on top.

4. Place on a baking sheet and bake for 15-20 minutes until bubbly.

Meal Prep: Best served fresh.

Time: 25 minutes

Nutritional Information:

- Calories: 90

- Fat: 7g

- Protein: 4g

- Carbs: 3g

Recipe 17: Tuna Cucumber Boats

Ingredients:

- Cucumbers

- Canned tuna

- Mayo or Greek yogurt

- Dill pickles

- Red onion

- Dijon mustard

Instructions:

1. Cut cucumbers in half lengthwise and scoop out seeds to form a 'boat.'

2. In a bowl, mix tuna, mayo or Greek yogurt, chopped pickles, red onion, and mustard.

3. Fill cucumber boats with the tuna mixture.

Meal Prep: Ideal for immediate consumption.

Time: 20 minutes

Nutritional Information:

- Calories: 130

- Fat: 6g

- Protein: 12g

- Carbs: 4g

Recipe 18: Cheddar Bacon Bites

Ingredients:

- Cheddar cheese cubes

- Bacon strips

Instructions:

1. Wrap each cheese cube with a slice of bacon.

2. Secure with a toothpick.

3. Bake in a preheated oven at 375°F (190°C) for 15-20 minutes or until bacon is crispy.

Meal Prep: Best served fresh.

Time: 25 minutes

Nutritional Information:

- Calories: 120

- Fat: 9g

- Protein: 8g

- Carbs: 2g

Recipe 19: Stuffed Mushrooms

Ingredients:

- Mushrooms

- Cream cheese

- Garlic

- Parmesan cheese

- Fresh parsley

Instructions:

1. Preheat the oven to 375°F (190°C).

2. Remove stems from mushrooms and place caps on a baking sheet.

3. Mix cream cheese, garlic, Parmesan, and parsley, then stuff the mushroom caps.

4. Bake for 15-20 minutes until mushrooms are tender.

Meal Prep: Best served fresh.

Time: 30 minutes

Nutritional Information:

- Calories: 110

- Fat: 8g

- Protein: 6g

- Carbs: 4g

DESSERTS RECIPES

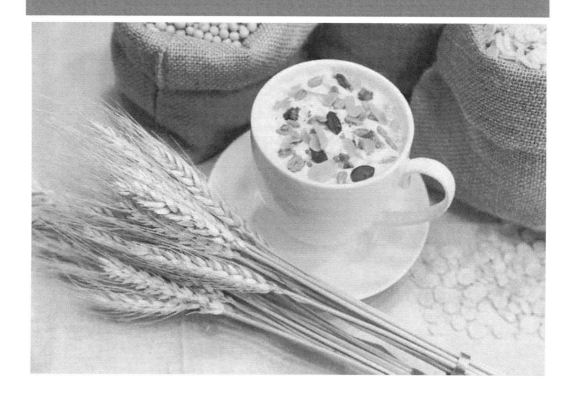

Recipe 1: Keto Chocolate Avocado Mousse

Ingredients:

- 2 ripe avocados

- 1/4 cup unsweetened cocoa powder

- 1/4 cup powdered erythritol

- 1 teaspoon vanilla extract

- 1/4 cup unsweetened almond milk

- Whipped cream (optional, for topping)

- Berries (optional, for garnish)

Instructions:

1. Peel and pit the avocados, placing them in a food processor or blender.

2. Add cocoa powder, erythritol, vanilla extract, and almond milk to the avocados.

3. Blend until smooth and creamy, scraping down the sides as needed.

4. Divide the mousse into serving dishes and chill in the refrigerator for at least an hour.

5. Top with whipped cream and berries if desired before serving.

Meal Prep:

- Prep Time: 10 minutes

- Total Time: 1 hour 10 minutes (including chilling)

- Yield: 4 servings

Nutritional Information (per serving):

- Calories: 180

- Fat: 15g

- Protein: 3g

- Carbohydrates: 10g

- Fiber: 7g

- Net Carbs: 3g

Recipe 2: Keto Lemon Cheesecake Bars

Ingredients:

- 2 cups almond flour

- 1/2 cup powdered erythritol

- 1/2 cup butter, melted

- 16 oz cream cheese, softened

- 2 large eggs

- 1/2 cup powdered erythritol (for cheesecake)

- Zest of 1 lemon

- Juice of 1 lemon

- 1 teaspoon vanilla extract

Instructions:

1. Preheat oven to 350°F (175°C) and line an 8x8-inch baking pan with parchment paper.

2. In a bowl, mix almond flour, 1/2 cup erythritol, and melted butter. Press into the bottom of the prepared pan.

3. Bake the crust for 12-15 minutes until lightly golden. Remove and let it cool.

4. In another bowl, beat cream cheese, eggs, 1/2 cup erythritol, lemon zest, lemon juice, and vanilla until smooth.

5. Pour the cheesecake mixture over the cooled crust.

6. Bake for 25-30 minutes until the edges are set and the center slightly jiggles.

7. Cool completely, then refrigerate for at least 3 hours before slicing into bars.

Meal Prep:

- Prep Time: 20 minutes

- Total Time: 4 hours 15 minutes (including chilling)

- Yield: 12 bars

Nutritional Information (per bar):

- Calories: 230

- Fat: 21g

- Protein: 5g

- Carbohydrates: 5g

- Fiber: 1g

- Net Carbs: 4g

Recipe 3: Keto Coconut Almond Fat Bombs

Ingredients:

- 1/2 cup almond butter

- 1/4 cup coconut oil, melted

- 2 tablespoons shredded unsweetened coconut

- 1 tablespoon powdered erythritol

- 1/2 teaspoon almond extract

- Pinch of salt

Instructions:

1. In a bowl, mix almond butter, melted coconut oil, shredded coconut, erythritol, almond extract, and a pinch of salt until well combined.

2. Using a small ice cream scoop or spoon, form the mixture into small balls and place on a parchment-lined tray.

3. Freeze for 20-30 minutes until firm.

4. Store in an airtight container in the refrigerator.

Meal Prep:

- Prep Time: 10 minutes

- Total Time: 30 minutes

- Yield: 12 fat bombs

Nutritional Information (per fat bomb):

- Calories: 90

- Fat: 9g

- Protein: 1g

- Carbohydrates: 2g

- Fiber: 1g

- Net Carbs: 1g

Recipe 4: Keto Raspberry Chia Seed Pudding

Ingredients:

1 cup unsweetened almond milk

- 1/4 cup chia seeds

- 1 tablespoon powdered erythritol

- 1/2 teaspoon vanilla extract

- 1/2 cup fresh raspberries

Instructions:

1. In a bowl, whisk together almond milk, chia seeds, erythritol, and vanilla extract.

2. Let the mixture sit for 10 minutes, then whisk again to break up any clumps.

3. Cover and refrigerate for at least 2 hours or overnight.

4. Before serving, layer the chia pudding and fresh raspberries in serving glasses or jars.

Meal Prep:

- Prep Time: 5 minutes

- Total Time: 2 hours 10 minutes

- Yield: 2 servings

Nutritional Information (per serving):

- Calories: 120

- Fat: 8g

- Protein: 3g

- Carbohydrates: 10g

- Fiber: 8g

- Net Carbs: 2g

Recipe 5: Keto Peanut Butter Chocolate Chip Cookies

Ingredients:

- 1 cup almond flour

- 1/2 cup powdered erythritol

- 1/2 cup unsweetened peanut butter

- 1/4 cup melted coconut oil

- 1 teaspoon vanilla extract

- 1/4 teaspoon baking soda

- 1/4 cup sugar-free chocolate chips

Instructions:

1. Preheat oven to 350°F (175°C) and line a baking sheet with parchment paper.

2. In a bowl, mix almond flour, erythritol, peanut butter,

melted coconut oil, vanilla extract, and baking soda until a dough forms.

3. Fold in the sugar-free chocolate chips.

4. Scoop dough onto the prepared baking sheet and flatten slightly with a fork.

5. Bake for 12-15 minutes until edges are golden.

6. Let the cookies cool on the sheet for 10 minutes before transferring to a wire rack to cool completely.

Meal Prep:

- Prep Time: 15 minutes

- Total Time: 30 minutes

- Yield: 12 cookies

Nutritional Information (per cookie):

- Calories: 160

- Fat: 14g

- Protein: 4g

- Carbohydrates: 5g

- Fiber: 2g

- Net Carbs: 3g

Recipe 6: Keto Blueberry Almond Flour Cake

Ingredients:

- 2 cups almond flour

- 1/2 cup powdered erythritol

- 1/4 cup melted butter

- 3 large eggs

- 1/4 cup unsweetened almond milk

- 1 teaspoon baking powder

- 1 teaspoon almond extract

- 1/2 cup fresh blueberries

Instructions:

1. Preheat oven to 350°F (175°C) and grease an 8-inch cake pan.

2. In a bowl, whisk together almond flour, erythritol, melted butter, eggs, almond milk, baking powder, and almond extract until smooth.

3. Gently fold in the fresh blueberries.

4. Pour the batter into the prepared cake pan.

5. Bake for 25-30 minutes until a toothpick inserted comes out clean.

6. Let the cake cool in the pan for 10 minutes, then transfer to a wire rack to cool completely.

Meal Prep:

- Prep Time: 15 minutes

- Total Time: 45 minutes

- Yield: 8 slices

Nutritional Information (per slice):

- Calories: 210

- Fat: 18g

- Protein: 7g

- Carbohydrates: 7g

- Fiber: 3g

- Net Carbs: 4g

Recipe 7: Keto Vanilla Coconut Macaroons

Ingredients:

- 3 cups shredded unsweetened coconut

- 1/2 cup powdered erythritol

- 3 egg whites

- 1 teaspoon vanilla extract

- 1/4 teaspoon salt

Instructions:

1. Preheat oven to 325°F (160°C) and line a baking sheet with parchment paper.

2. In a bowl, mix together shredded coconut, erythritol,

egg whites, vanilla extract, and salt until well combined.

3. Using a cookie scoop or spoon, form the mixture into mounds on the prepared baking sheet.

4. Bake for 20-25 minutes until the edges are golden.

5. Cool completely on the baking sheet before removing.

Meal Prep:

- Prep Time: 10 minutes

- Total Time: 35 minutes

- Yield: 18 macaroons

Nutritional Information (per macaroon):

- Calories: 80

- Fat: 7g

- Protein: 2g

- Carbohydrates: 4g

- Fiber: 2g

- Net Carbs: 2g

Recipe 8: Keto Chocolate Peanut Butter Fat Bombs

Ingredients:

- 1/2 cup unsweetened peanut butter

- 1/4 cup coconut oil, melted

- 2 tablespoons unsweetened cocoa powder

- 2 tablespoons powdered erythritol

- 1/2 teaspoon vanilla extract

Instructions:

1. In a bowl, mix peanut butter, melted coconut oil, cocoa powder, erythritol, and vanilla extract until smooth.

2. Pour the mixture into silicone molds or lined mini muffin tins.

3. Freeze for 30-40 minutes until firm.

4. Store in an airtight container in the refrigerator.

Meal Prep:

- Prep Time: 10 minutes

- Total Time: 40 minutes

- Yield: 12 fat bombs

Nutritional Information (per fat bomb):

- Calories: 90

- Fat: 8g

- Protein: 2g

- Carbohydrates: 3g

- Fiber: 2g

- Net Carbs: 1g

Recipe 9: Keto Pumpkin Spice Fat Bombs

Ingredients:

- 1/2 cup pumpkin puree

- 1/4 cup coconut oil, melted

- 2 tablespoons powdered erythritol

- 1 teaspoon pumpkin pie spice

- 1/2 teaspoon vanilla extract

- Chopped pecans (optional, for topping)

Instructions:

1. In a bowl, mix pumpkin puree, melted coconut oil, erythritol, pumpkin pie spice, and vanilla extract until well combined.

2. Pour the mixture into silicone molds or lined mini muffin tins.

3. Top with chopped pecans if desired.

4. Freeze for 30-40 minutes until firm.

5. Store in an airtight container in the refrigerator.

Meal Prep:

- Prep Time: 10 minutes

- Total Time: 40 minutes

- Yield: 12 fat bombs

Nutritional Information (per fat bomb):

- Calories: 60

- Fat: 6g

- Protein: 1g

- Carbohydrates: 2g

- Fiber: 1g

- Net Carbs: 1g

Recipe 10: Keto Strawberry Cream Cheese Fat Bombs

Ingredients:

- 4 oz cream cheese, softened

- 1/4 cup coconut oil, melted

- 2 tablespoons powdered erythritol

- 1/4 cup chopped strawberries

- 1/2 teaspoon vanilla extract

Instructions:

1. In a bowl, beat cream cheese, melted coconut oil, erythritol, strawberries, and vanilla extract until smooth.

2. Pour the mixture into silicone molds or lined mini muffin tins.

3. Freeze for 30-40 minutes until firm.

4. Store in an airtight container in the refrigerator.

Meal Prep:

- Prep Time: 10 minutes

- Total Time: 40 minutes

- Yield: 12 fat bombs

Nutritional Information (per fat bomb):

- Calories: 70

- Fat: 7g

- Protein: 1g

- Carbohydrates: 1g

- Fiber: 0g

- Net Carbs: 1g

Recipe 11: Keto Chocolate Chia Pudding

Ingredients:

- 1 cup unsweetened almond milk

- 1/4 cup chia seeds

- 2 tablespoons unsweetened cocoa powder

- 2 tablespoons powdered erythritol

- 1/2 teaspoon vanilla extract

Instructions:

1. In a bowl, whisk together almond milk, chia seeds, cocoa powder, erythritol, and vanilla extract.

2. Let the mixture sit for 10 minutes, then whisk again to break up any clumps.

3. Cover and refrigerate for at least 2 hours or overnight.

4. Stir well before serving.

Meal Prep:

- Prep Time: 5 minutes

- Total Time: 2 hours 10 minutes

- Yield: 2 servings

Nutritional Information (per serving):

- Calories: 130

- Fat: 9g

- Protein: 4g

- Carbohydrates: 10g

- Fiber: 7g

- Net Carbs: 3g

AIR FRYER RECIPES

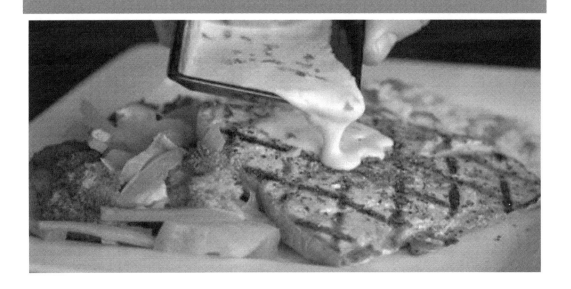

Recipe 1: Crispy Parmesan Chicken Tenders

Ingredients:

- 1 pound chicken tenders
- 1/2 cup grated Parmesan cheese
- 1/4 cup almond flour
- 1 teaspoon paprika
- 1 teaspoon garlic powder
- Salt and pepper to taste

- 2 beaten eggs

Instructions:

1. Preheat the air fryer to 375°F.

2. In a shallow dish, mix Parmesan, almond flour, paprika, garlic powder, salt, and pepper.

3. Dip chicken tenders in beaten eggs, then coat with the Parmesan mixture.

4. Place tenders in the air fryer basket in a single layer.

5. Air fry for 10-12 minutes, flipping halfway through.

Meal Prep: Serve with a side of keto-friendly dipping sauce and a green salad.

Preparation Time: 20 minutes
Nutritional Information: (Per serving)
Calories: 280
Fat: 15g
Protein: 30g
Carbohydrates: 3g

Recipe 2: Zesty Lemon Pepper Salmon

Ingredients:

- 4 salmon fillets

- 2 tablespoons olive oil

- 1 teaspoon lemon zest

- 1 teaspoon black pepper

- 1 teaspoon dried parsley

- 1/2 teaspoon garlic powder

- Salt to taste

- Lemon wedges for garnish

Instructions:

1. Preheat the air fryer to 400°F.

2. Rub salmon fillets with olive oil and season with lemon zest, black pepper, parsley, garlic powder, and salt.

3. Place the fillets in the air fryer basket.

4. Air fry for 8-10 minutes until the salmon is cooked through.

Meal Prep: Serve with steamed vegetables or a side of cauliflower rice.

Preparation Time: 15 minutes
Nutritional Information: (Per serving)
Calories: 320
Fat: 20g

Protein: 35g

Carbohydrates: 1g

Recipe 3: Crispy Garlic Parmesan Brussels Sprouts

Ingredients:

- 1 pound Brussels sprouts, halved

- 2 tablespoons olive oil

- 1/4 cup grated Parmesan cheese

- 2 cloves minced garlic

- 1 teaspoon Italian seasoning

- Salt and pepper to taste

Instructions:

1. Preheat the air fryer to 375°F.

2. In a bowl, toss Brussels sprouts with olive oil, Parmesan, garlic, Italian seasoning, salt, and pepper.

3. Place the seasoned sprouts in the air fryer basket.

4. Air fry for 12-15 minutes, shaking the basket halfway through.

Meal Prep: Enjoy as a tasty side dish with your favorite protein.

Preparation Time: 20 minutes
Nutritional Information: (Per serving)
Calories: 120
Fat: 7g
Protein: 5g
Carbohydrates: 10g

Recipe 4: Crispy Coconut Shrimp

Ingredients:

- 1 pound large shrimp, peeled and deveined

- 1/2 cup shredded unsweetened coconut

- 1/4 cup almond flour

- 2 beaten eggs

- Salt and pepper to taste

- Lime wedges for serving

Instructions:

1. Preheat the air fryer to 400°F.

2. In one bowl, mix coconut and almond flour. In another bowl, place beaten eggs.

3. Dip shrimp in the egg, then coat with the coconut mixture.

4. Place the coated shrimp in the air fryer basket.

5. Air fry for 8-10 minutes, flipping once.

Meal Prep: Serve as an appetizer or with a side of mixed greens.

Preparation Time: 25 minutes
Nutritional Information: (Per serving)
Calories: 220
Fat: 14g
Protein: 20g
Carbohydrates: 5g

Recipe 5: Spicy Cajun Pork Chops

Ingredients:

- 4 pork chops

- 2 tablespoons Cajun seasoning

- 1 tablespoon olive oil

- 1 teaspoon smoked paprika

- 1/2 teaspoon cayenne pepper

- Salt and pepper to taste

Instructions:

1. Preheat the air fryer to 380°F.

2. Rub pork chops with Cajun seasoning, olive oil, paprika, cayenne, salt, and pepper.

3. Place the seasoned chops in the air fryer basket.

4. Air fry for 12-15 minutes, flipping halfway through.

Meal Prep: Pair with a side of sautéed spinach or roasted asparagus.

Preparation Time: 18 minutes
Nutritional Information: (Per

serving)

Calories: 280

Fat: 16g

Protein: 30g

Carbohydrates: 2g

Recipe 6: Herb-Roasted Chicken Thighs

Ingredients:

- 6 bone-in, skin-on chicken thighs

- 2 tablespoons olive oil

- 1 teaspoon dried thyme

- 1 teaspoon dried rosemary

- 1 teaspoon garlic powder

- Salt and pepper to taste

Instructions:

1. Preheat the air fryer to 380°F.

2. Rub chicken thighs with olive oil, thyme, rosemary, garlic powder, salt, and pepper.

3. Place the seasoned thighs in the air fryer basket, skin side up.

4. Air fry for 25-30 minutes until golden and cooked through.

Meal Prep: Serve with a side of roasted vegetables or a fresh salad.

Preparation Time: 30 minutes
Nutritional Information: (Per serving)

Calories: 320

Fat: 22g

Protein: 28g

Carbohydrates: 1g

Recipe 7: Savory Garlic Green Beans

Ingredients:

- 1 pound fresh green beans, trimmed

- 2 tablespoons butter

- 3 cloves minced garlic

- 1/4 cup sliced almonds

- Salt and pepper to taste

Instructions:

1. Preheat the air fryer to 375°F.

2. In a bowl, toss green beans with butter, garlic, almonds, salt, and pepper.

3. Place the seasoned green beans in the air fryer basket.

4. Air fry for 10-12 minutes, shaking the basket occasionally.

Meal Prep: Enjoy as a side with grilled chicken or steak.

Preparation Time: 15 minutes
Nutritional Information: (Per serving)
Calories: 110
Fat: 8g
Protein: 3g
Carbohydrates: 8g

Recipe 8: Lemon-Garlic Asparagus Spears

Ingredients:

- 1 bunch asparagus, trimmed

- 2 tablespoons olive oil

- Zest of 1 lemon

- 2 cloves minced garlic

- Salt and pepper to taste

Instructions:

1. Preheat the air fryer to 400°F.

2. Toss asparagus with olive oil, lemon zest, garlic, salt, and pepper in a bowl.

3. Place the seasoned asparagus in the air fryer basket.

4. Air fry for 8-10 minutes until tender-crisp.

Meal Prep: Pair with a grilled protein of your choice or enjoy as a light snack.

Preparation Time: 12 minutes
Nutritional Information: (Per serving)
Calories: 90

Fat: 7g

Protein: 4g

Carbohydrates: 6g

Recipe 9: Crispy Bacon-Wrapped Asparagus

Ingredients:

- 12 asparagus spears

- 6 slices bacon

- Salt and black pepper to taste

Instructions:

1. Preheat the air fryer to 390°F.

2. Wrap each asparagus spear with half a slice of bacon, season with salt and pepper.

3. Place the bacon-wrapped asparagus in the air fryer basket.

4. Air fry for 10-12 minutes until the bacon is crispy.

Meal Prep: Serve as an appetizer or alongside a main dish for added flavor.

Preparation Time: 15 minutes

Nutritional Information: (Per serving)

Calories: 120

Fat: 9g

Protein: 5g

Carbohydrates: 3g

Recipe 10: Cajun Lime Avocado Fries

Ingredients:

- 2 ripe avocados, sliced into wedges

- 1/2 cup almond flour

- 2 teaspoons Cajun seasoning

- Zest of 1 lime

- 2 beaten eggs

Instructions:

1. Preheat the air fryer to 375°F.

2. In a bowl, mix almond flour, Cajun seasoning, and lime zest.

3. Dip avocado slices in beaten eggs, then coat with the almond flour mixture.

4. Place the avocado fries in the air fryer basket.

5. Air fry for 6-8 minutes until golden and crispy.

Meal Prep: Enjoy as a snack or appetizer with a side of salsa or dip.

Preparation Time: 20 minutes
Nutritional Information: (Per serving)
Calories: 160
Fat: 12g
Protein: 3g
Carbohydrates: 10g

Recipe 11: Garlic Herb Mushrooms

Ingredients:

- 1 pound whole mushrooms, cleaned

- 2 tablespoons olive oil

- 2 cloves minced garlic

- 1 teaspoon dried thyme

- 1 teaspoon dried parsley

- Salt and pepper to taste

Instructions:

1. Preheat the air fryer to 380°F.

2. In a bowl, toss mushrooms with olive oil, garlic, thyme, parsley, salt, and pepper.

3. Place the seasoned mushrooms in the air fryer basket.

4. Air fry for 12-15 minutes, shaking occasionally.

Meal Prep: Serve as a side dish or as a topping for grilled meats.

Preparation Time: 18 minutes
Nutritional Information: (Per serving)
Calories: 90
Fat: 7g
Protein: 3g
Carbohydrates: 5g

Recipe 12: Crispy Garlic-Parmesan Zucchini Chips

Ingredients:

- 2 medium zucchinis, sliced into rounds

- 1/2 cup grated Parmesan cheese

- 1/4 cup almond flour

- 1 teaspoon garlic powder

- Salt and pepper to taste

- 2 beaten eggs

Instructions:

1. Preheat the air fryer to 380°F.

2. In a shallow dish, combine Parmesan, almond flour, garlic powder, salt, and pepper.

3. Dip zucchini slices in beaten eggs, then coat with the Parmesan mixture.

4. Place the coated zucchini in the air fryer basket.

5. Air fry for 8-10 minutes until golden and crisp.

Meal Prep: Enjoy as a guilt-free snack or as a side with a main dish.

Preparation Time: 22 minutes
Nutritional Information: (Per serving)
Calories: 120
Fat: 8g
Protein: 6g
Carbohydrates: 8g

Recipe 13: Lemon-Garlic Chicken Wings

Ingredients:

- 2 pounds chicken wings

- 2 tablespoons olive oil

- Zest of 1 lemon

- 2 cloves minced garlic

- 1 teaspoon dried thyme

- Salt and pepper to taste

Instructions:

1. Preheat the air fryer to 380°F.

2. Toss chicken wings with olive oil, lemon zest, garlic, thyme, salt, and pepper in a bowl.

3. Place the seasoned wings in the air fryer basket.

4. Air fry for 25-30 minutes, flipping halfway through.

Meal Prep: Perfect for a game day snack or as part of a dinner spread.

Preparation Time: 35 minutes
Nutritional Information: (Per serving)

Calories: 240
Fat: 16g
Protein: 20g
Carbohydrates: 1g

Recipe 14: Parmesan-Crusted Pork Tenderloin

Ingredients:

- 1 pork tenderloin
- 1/2 cup grated Parmesan cheese
- 1/4 cup almond flour
- 1 teaspoon dried oregano
- 1 teaspoon garlic powder
- Salt and pepper to taste

Instructions:

1. Preheat the air fryer to 400°F.

2. In a shallow dish, mix Parmesan, almond flour, oregano, garlic powder, salt, and pepper.

3. Coat the pork tenderloin with the Parmesan mixture.

4. Place the coated tenderloin in the air fryer basket.

5. Air fry for 20-25 minutes until internal temperature reaches 145°F.

Meal Prep: Serve with roasted vegetables for a wholesome meal.

Preparation Time: 30 minutes

Nutritional Information: (Per serving)

Calories: 280

Fat: 12g

Protein: 35g

Carbohydrates: 2g

Recipe 15: Turmeric-Spiced Cauliflower Bites

Ingredients:

- 1 head cauliflower, cut into florets

- 2 tablespoons olive oil

- 1 teaspoon turmeric

- 1 teaspoon cumin

- 1/2 teaspoon smoked paprika

- Salt and pepper to taste

Instructions:

1. Preheat the air fryer to 375°F.

2. Toss cauliflower with olive oil, turmeric, cumin, paprika, salt, and pepper in a bowl.

3. Place the seasoned cauliflower in the air fryer basket.

4. Air fry for 15-18 minutes until golden and tender.

Meal Prep: Enjoy as a flavorful side dish or a healthy snack.

Preparation Time: 25 minutes

Nutritional Information: (Per serving)

Calories: 90

Fat: 6g

Protein: 3g

Carbohydrates: 9g

KETO RECIPES FOR SPECIFIC DIETARY NEEDS (E.G., VEGETARIAN, VEGAN, GLUTEN-FREE, ETC.)

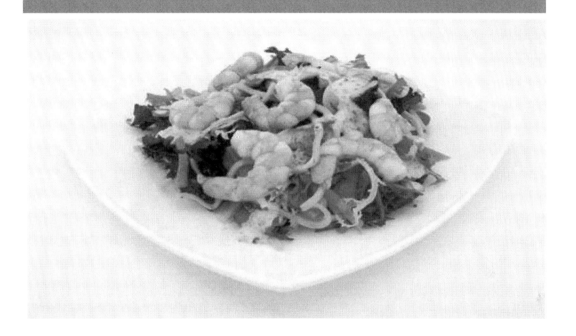

1. Vegetarian Zucchini Noodles with Pesto

Ingredients:

- 2 medium zucchinis

- 1 cup fresh basil leaves

- 1/4 cup pine nuts

- 2 cloves garlic

- 1/2 cup grated Parmesan cheese

- 1/4 cup olive oil

- Salt and pepper to taste

Instructions:

1. Spiralize the zucchinis into noodle shapes.

2. In a food processor, blend basil, pine nuts, garlic, and Parmesan. Slowly add olive oil until smooth.

3. Toss zucchini noodles with pesto, season with salt and pepper.

Meal Prep: Takes 20 minutes to prepare. Perfect for a quick lunch or light dinner.

Nutritional Information:

- Calories: 210

- Carbs: 6g

- Protein: 5g

- Fat: 18g

2. Gluten-Free Cauliflower Crust Pizza

Ingredients:

- 1 small cauliflower head

- 1 egg

- 1/2 cup shredded mozzarella

- 1/2 teaspoon dried oregano

- 1/4 teaspoon garlic powder

- Toppings of your choice (tomato sauce, cheese, veggies)

Instructions:

1. Rice cauliflower and microwave for 4 minutes. Let it cool, then squeeze excess moisture using a cloth.

2. Mix cauliflower, egg, mozzarella, oregano, and garlic powder, spread into a circle on a baking sheet.

3. Bake at 400°F for 20 mins. Add toppings and bake for an extra 10 mins.

Meal Prep: Prep time is around 30 minutes. Great for a weekend dinner.

Nutritional Information:

- Calories: 210

- Carbs: 8g

- Protein: 15g

- Fat: 14g

3. Vegan Avocado and Cucumber Soup

Ingredients:

- 2 ripe avocados

- 1 cucumber, peeled and seeded

- 2 cups vegetable broth

- 1/4 cup fresh cilantro

- Juice of 1 lime

- Salt and pepper to taste

Instructions:

1. Blend avocados, cucumber, vegetable broth, cilantro, and lime juice until smooth.

2. Season with salt and pepper.

3. Chill for at least 1 hour before serving.

Meal Prep: Preparation time is about 15 minutes. Ideal for a refreshing lunch option.

Nutritional Information:

- Calories: 180

- Carbs: 12g

- Protein: 4g

- Fat: 15g

4. Gluten-Free Eggplant Parmesan

Ingredients:

- 1 large eggplant

- 1 cup almond flour

- 2 eggs

- 1 cup marinara sauce

- 1 cup shredded mozzarella cheese

- 1/4 cup grated Parmesan cheese

- Fresh basil for garnish

Instructions:

1. Slice eggplant, dip in beaten eggs, then coat with almond flour. Bake at 400°F for 20 minutes.

2. Layer eggplant slices in a baking dish, top with marinara and cheeses. Bake for an additional 15 minutes.

3. Garnish with fresh basil.

Meal Prep: Approximately 45 minutes for preparation. Perfect for a cozy dinner.

Nutritional Information:

- Calories: 280

- Carbs: 15g

- Protein: 14g

- Fat: 20g

5. Vegetarian Cauliflower Fried Rice

Ingredients:

- 1 head cauliflower

- 2 tablespoons sesame oil

- 1 cup mixed vegetables (peas, carrots, bell peppers)

- 2 eggs, beaten

- 3 tablespoons soy sauce or tamari

- Green onions for garnish

Instructions:

1. Rice cauliflower using a food processor.

2. In a pan, heat sesame oil, add mixed vegetables, and stir-fry for a few minutes.

3. Push veggies to the side, scramble eggs, then mix with vegetables and add cauliflower rice. Stir in soy sauce.

4. Garnish with green onions.

Meal Prep: Prep time is about 25 minutes. Great for a quick weeknight dinner.

Nutritional Information:

- Calories: 230
- Carbs: 12g
- Protein: 10g
- Fat: 16g

6. Vegan Coconut Curry with Tofu

Ingredients:

- 1 block firm tofu, cubed
- 1 tablespoon coconut oil
- 1 onion, diced
- 2 cloves garlic, minced
- 1 can coconut milk
- 2 tablespoons curry powder
- Salt and pepper to taste
- Fresh cilantro for garnish

Instructions:

1. Sauté onion and garlic in coconut oil until soft. Add tofu, cook until lightly browned.

2. Pour in coconut milk, curry powder, salt, and pepper. Simmer for 10-15 minutes.

3. Serve with fresh cilantro.

Meal Prep: Takes around 30 minutes to prepare. A flavorful dinner option.

Nutritional Information:

- Calories: 320
- Carbs: 10g
- Protein: 15g
- Fat: 25g

7. Gluten-Free Portobello Mushroom Burger

Ingredients:

- 4 large portobello mushroom caps

- 1/4 cup balsamic vinegar

- 2 tablespoons olive oil

- 1 teaspoon dried basil

- Salt and pepper to taste

- Lettuce, tomatoes, and your choice of toppings

Instructions:

1. Mix balsamic vinegar, olive oil, basil, salt, and pepper. Marinate mushroom caps for 30 mins.

2. Grill mushrooms for 4-5 minutes on each side.

3. Assemble burgers using lettuce, tomatoes, and preferred toppings.

Meal Prep: Preparation time is around 40 minutes. Perfect for a BBQ or weekend lunch.

Nutritional Information:

- Calories: 180

- Carbs: 10g

- Protein: 6g

- Fat: 12g

8. Vegetarian Caprese Stuffed Avocados

Ingredients:

- 2 ripe avocados

- 1 cup cherry tomatoes, halved

- 1/2 cup fresh mozzarella balls, halved

- 2 tablespoons balsamic glaze

- Fresh basil leaves

- Salt and pepper to taste

Instructions:

1. Cut avocados in half and remove pits. Scoop out some flesh to create space.

2. In a bowl, mix tomatoes, mozzarella, balsamic glaze, basil, salt, and pepper. Stuff avocados with the mixture.

Meal Prep: Prep time is around 15 minutes. Ideal for a quick and healthy lunch.

Nutritional Information:

- Calories: 250

- Carbs: 10g

- Protein: 8g

- Fat: 20g

9. Gluten-Free Cauliflower Mac and Cheese

Ingredients:

- 1 head cauliflower

- 1 cup heavy cream

- 1 cup shredded cheddar cheese

- 1/4 cup grated Parmesan cheese

- 1/2 teaspoon mustard powder

- Salt and pepper to taste

Instructions:

1. Steam cauliflower until tender, then blend until smooth.

2. In a pot, heat heavy cream, add cheddar, Parmesan, mustard powder, salt, and pepper. Stir until cheese melts.

3. Mix cheese sauce with cauliflower puree.

Meal Prep: Takes about 25 minutes to prepare. Perfect for a cozy dinner.

Nutritional Information:

- Calories: 280

- Carbs: 10g

- Protein: 12g

- Fat: 22g

10. Vegan Spaghetti Squash Pad Thai

Ingredients:

- 1 large spaghetti squash
- 1 tablespoon sesame oil
- 1 bell pepper, julienned
- 1 cup bean sprouts
- 1/4 cup chopped peanuts
- 2 tablespoons soy sauce or tamari
- Lime wedges for serving

Instructions:

1. Roast spaghetti squash until tender, scrape into "noodles."
2. In a pan, heat sesame oil, add bell pepper and bean sprouts. Stir-fry for a few minutes.
3. Add spaghetti squash, soy sauce, and toss together.
4. Top with chopped peanuts and serve with lime wedges.

Meal Prep: Prep time is about 35 minutes. Great for a flavorful dinner.

Nutritional Information:

- Calories: 240
- Carbs: 15g
- Protein: 8g
- Fat: 18g

11. Gluten-Free Broccoli Cheddar Soup

Ingredients:

- 2 cups broccoli florets
- 2 cups vegetable broth
- 1 cup heavy cream
- 1 cup shredded cheddar cheese
- 2 tablespoons butter
- Salt and pepper to taste

Instructions:

1. Steam broccoli until tender.
2. In a pot, combine broth, heavy cream, cheddar, butter, salt,

and pepper. Stir over medium heat until cheese melts.

3. Blend broccoli and add to the soup, simmer for a few minutes.

Meal Prep: Takes around 30 minutes to prepare. Perfect for a comforting dinner.

Nutritional Information:

- Calories: 260

- Carbs: 8g

- Protein: 10g

- Fat: 20g

12. Vegetarian Keto Stuffed Bell Peppers

Ingredients:

- 4 bell peppers

- 1 cup cauliflower rice

- 1 cup black beans

- 1 cup shredded cheddar cheese

- 1/2 cup salsa

- Fresh cilantro for garnish

- Salt and pepper to taste

Instructions:

1. Cut the tops off bell peppers, remove seeds.

2. Mix cauliflower rice, black beans, 3/4 cup cheese, salsa, salt, and pepper. Stuff into peppers.

3. Top with remaining cheese, bake at 375°F for 25 minutes.

4. Garnish with fresh cilantro.

Meal Prep: Preparation time is around 40 minutes. Ideal for a filling dinner.

Nutritional Information:

- Calories: 290

- Carbs: 18g

- Protein: 12g

- Fat: 18g

13. Vegan Keto Stir-Fry Tofu with Vegetables

Ingredients:

- 1 block firm tofu, cubed

- 2 tablespoons olive oil

- 2 cups mixed vegetables (broccoli, bell peppers, snow peas)

- 2 tablespoons soy sauce or tamari

- 1 teaspoon sesame seeds

Instructions:

1. Sauté tofu in olive oil until lightly browned. Remove from pan.

2. Stir-fry vegetables in the same pan, add tofu back in, drizzle with soy sauce, and cook for a few more minutes.

3. Garnish with sesame seeds.

Meal Prep: Prep time is about 25 minutes. Great for a quick and tasty dinner.

Nutritional Information:

- Calories: 260

- Carbs: 10g

- Protein: 15g

- Fat: 18g

14. Gluten-Free Veggie Cauliflower Crust Pizza

Ingredients:

- 1 small cauliflower head

- 1 egg

- 1/2 cup shredded mozzarella

- 1/2 teaspoon dried oregano

- Toppings of choice (sliced tomatoes, bell peppers, onions)

Instructions:

1. Rice cauliflower and microwave for 4 minutes. Let it cool, then squeeze excess moisture using a cloth.

2. Mix cauliflower, egg, mozzarella, and oregano, spread into a circle on a baking sheet.

3. Bake at 400°F for 20 mins. Add toppings and bake for an extra 10 mins.

Meal Prep: Prep time is about 30 minutes. Perfect for a satisfying dinner.

Nutritional Information:

- Calories: 220

- Carbs: 10g

- Protein: 14g

- Fat: 16g

15. Vegetarian Keto Broccoli Cheddar Casserole

Ingredients:

- 4 cups steamed broccoli florets

- 1 cup heavy cream

- 1 cup shredded cheddar cheese

- 2 tablespoons almond flour

- 2 tablespoons butter

- Salt and pepper to taste

Instructions:

1. Mix steamed broccoli, heavy cream, cheddar, almond flour, butter, salt, and pepper in a casserole dish.

2. Bake at 375°F for 25 minutes until bubbly and golden on top.

Meal Prep: Takes around 35 minutes to prepare. Ideal for a comforting dinner.

Nutritional Information:

- Calories: 280

- Carbs: 12g

- Protein: 10g

- Fat: 20g

16. Vegan Keto Coconut Curry Vegetables

Ingredients:

- 2 cups mixed vegetables (cauliflower, bell peppers, carrots)
- 1 can coconut milk
- 2 tablespoons curry powder
- 1 tablespoon coconut oil
- Salt and pepper to taste
- Fresh cilantro for garnish

Instructions:

1. Sauté mixed vegetables in coconut oil until slightly tender.
2. Pour in coconut milk, curry powder, salt, and pepper. Simmer for 15 minutes.
3. Garnish with fresh cilantro.

Meal Prep: Prep time is about 30 minutes. Great for a flavorful dinner.

Nutritional Information:

- Calories: 240
- Carbs: 12g
- Protein: 8g
- Fat: 15g

28-DAYS MEAL PLAN

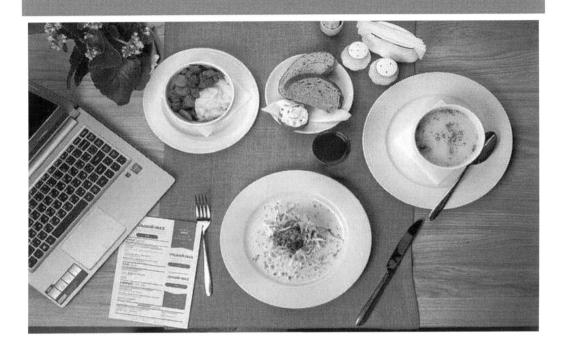

WEEK 1

Day 1:

- Breakfast: Scrambled eggs with spinach and avocado

- Lunch: Grilled chicken salad with mixed greens, olive oil, and nuts

- Dinner: Baked salmon with roasted asparagus

Day 2:

- Breakfast: Keto chia seed pudding

- Lunch: Zucchini noodles with pesto and grilled shrimp

- Dinner: Beef stir-fry with broccoli and cauliflower rice

Day 3:

- Breakfast: Keto smoothie (almond milk, berries, spinach, and protein powder)

- Lunch: Turkey lettuce wraps with avocado and salsa

- Dinner: Grilled lamb chops with steamed green beans

Day 4:

- Breakfast: Keto pancakes with sugar-free syrup

- Lunch: Tuna salad stuffed in bell peppers

- Dinner: Baked chicken thighs with a side of sautéed kale

Day 5:

- Breakfast: Avocado and bacon omelette

- Lunch: Cauliflower crust pizza with vegetables and cheese

- Dinner: Pork tenderloin with roasted Brussels sprouts

Day 6:

- Breakfast: Coconut flour muffins with sugar-free jam

- Lunch: Egg salad with mixed greens

- Dinner: Pan-seared cod with a side of roasted cauliflower

Day 7:

- Breakfast: Keto-friendly yogurt with nuts and seeds

- Lunch: Shredded chicken salad with avocado and a vinaigrette dressing

- Dinner: Grilled steak with a side of sautéed spinach

WEEK 2

Day 8:

- Breakfast: Spinach and feta omelette

- Lunch: Chicken Caesar salad with a keto-friendly dressing

- Dinner: Baked halibut with roasted vegetables

Day 9:

- Breakfast: Keto coconut flour porridge

- Lunch: Tofu and vegetable stir-fry with cauliflower rice

- Dinner: Grilled turkey burgers with a side of steamed broccoli

Day 10:

- Breakfast: Keto-friendly muffins with sugar-free cream cheese

- Lunch: Shrimp and avocado salad with a lemon vinaigrette

- Dinner: Beef kebabs with grilled bell peppers and onions

Day 11:

- Breakfast: Keto smoothie bowl with coconut and berries

- Lunch: Eggplant lasagna with a side salad

- Dinner: Roast chicken with sautéed spinach

Day 12:

- Breakfast: Chaffles (cheese waffles) with sugar-free syrup

- Lunch: Greek salad with grilled chicken

- Dinner: Baked cod with a side of roasted asparagus

Day 13:

- Breakfast: Keto crustless quiche with spinach and bacon

- Lunch: Tuna and avocado salad in lettuce wraps

- Dinner: Pork loin chops with steamed green beans

Day 14:

- Breakfast: Almond flour pancakes with berries

- Lunch: Cobb salad with grilled steak

- Dinner: Baked salmon with a side of cauliflower mash

WEEK 3

Day 15:

- Breakfast: Scrambled eggs with smoked salmon and avocado

- Lunch: Grilled chicken Caesar salad

- Dinner: Baked turkey meatballs with zucchini noodles

Day 16:

- Breakfast: Keto blueberry muffins

- Lunch: Tuna salad stuffed in avocado halves

- Dinner: Pan-seared shrimp with garlic butter over cauliflower rice

Day 17:

- Breakfast: Spinach and mushroom frittata

- Lunch: Cobb salad with grilled chicken and avocado

- Dinner: Herb-roasted pork tenderloin with roasted Brussels sprouts

Day 18:

- Breakfast: Keto cinnamon roll smoothie

- Lunch: Egg salad lettuce wraps

- Dinner: Baked cod with a side of sautéed kale

Day 19:

- Breakfast: Almond flour waffles with sugar-free syrup

- Lunch: Grilled steak salad with mixed greens

- Dinner: Lemon herb chicken with steamed broccoli

Day 20:

- Breakfast: Keto-friendly bagels with cream cheese

- Lunch: Zucchini noodles with pesto and grilled shrimp

- Dinner: Beef stir-fry with cauliflower rice

Day 21:

- Breakfast: Keto pancakes with berries and whipped cream

- Lunch: Greek salad with grilled chicken

- Dinner: Baked salmon with roasted asparagus

WEEK 4

Day 22:

- Breakfast: Keto chia seed pudding with sliced almonds

- Lunch: Chicken and avocado salad with a low-carb dressing

- Dinner: Grilled lamb chops with a side of roasted vegetables

Day 23:

- Breakfast: Spinach and feta crustless quiche

- Lunch: Tuna salad lettuce wraps with sliced cucumbers

- Dinner: Baked chicken thighs with sautéed spinach

Day 24:

- Breakfast: Keto smoothie with avocado and cocoa powder

- Lunch: Shrimp and zucchini noodles with garlic and olive oil

- Dinner: Beef and broccoli stir-fry with cauliflower rice

Day 25:

- Breakfast: Keto coconut flour pancakes with sugar-free syrup

- Lunch: Greek salad with grilled chicken

- Dinner: Baked salmon with a side of roasted asparagus

Day 26:

- Breakfast: Almond flour waffles with fresh berries

- Lunch: Turkey lettuce wraps with avocado and salsa

- Dinner: Pork tenderloin with steamed green beans

Day 27:

- Breakfast: Keto crustless quiche with spinach and bacon

- Lunch: Egg salad with mixed greens

- Dinner: Pan-seared cod with a side of roasted cauliflower

Day 28:

- Breakfast: Scrambled eggs with diced tomatoes and avocado

- Lunch: Cobb salad with grilled steak

- Dinner: Baked chicken with a side of sautéed kale

This 28-day meal plan aims to provide a varied and nutrient-rich selection of ketogenic meals that might be considered by some individuals dealing with health conditions such as cancer. Always consult with a healthcare professional or a registered dietitian before making significant dietary changes, particularly if you're managing health concerns.

Please adapt the meal plan to suit individual dietary needs and preferences. Keeping track of how your body responds to the diet and making adjustments accordingly is crucial. It's also essential to prioritize whole, nutrient-dense foods while following a ketogenic diet for health-related purposes.

This plan is a general guide and should be personalized based on specific health conditions, dietary requirements, and professional guidance.

Always prioritize your health and well-being above following a strict meal plan, and make adjustments based on how your body responds to the diet.

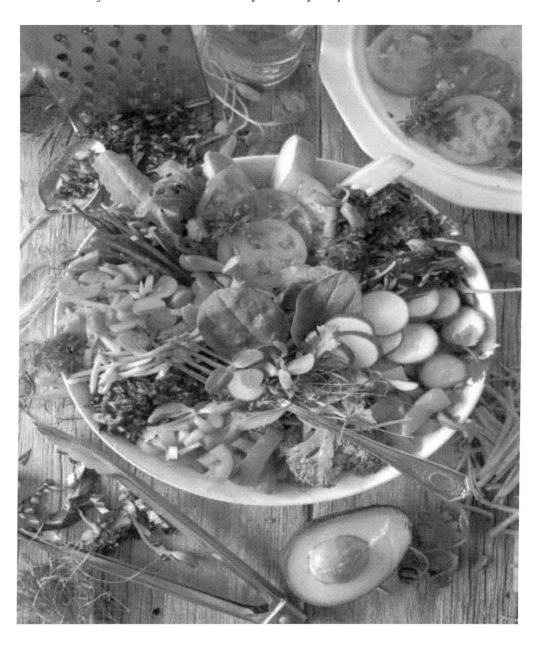

NUTRITIONAL SUPPLEMENTS FOR CANCER PATIENTS ON THE KETOGENIC DIET

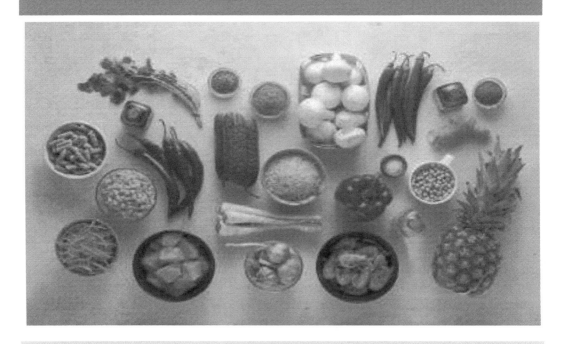

WHICH NUTRITIONAL SUPPLEMENTS ARE BENEFICIAL FOR CANCER PATIENTS ON THE KETOGENIC DIET?

There are a number of nutritional supplements that may be beneficial for cancer patients on the ketogenic diet. Some of the most well-studied supplements include:

- MCT oil: MCT oil is a type of fat that is easily digested and converted into ketones. It may help to improve energy levels and reduce side effects of the ketogenic diet, such as fatigue and nausea.

- Omega-3 fatty acids: Omega-3 fatty acids have anti-inflammatory and anti-cancer properties. They may help to reduce the risk of cancer progression and improve overall survival.

- Glutamine: Glutamine is an amino acid that is essential for gut health. It may help to reduce the risk of intestinal damage and infection, which can be common in cancer patients.

- Electrolytes: Electrolytes, such as sodium, potassium, and magnesium, are important for maintaining fluid balance and muscle function. They may be lost in the urine during the ketogenic diet, so it is important to supplement with them.

- Multivitamin: A multivitamin can help to ensure that you are getting all of the essential vitamins and minerals that your body needs, especially if you are following a restrictive diet such as the ketogenic diet.

OTHER SUPPLEMENTS THAT MAY BE BENEFICIAL FOR CANCER PATIENTS ON THE KETOGENIC DIET INCLUDE:

- Probiotics: Probiotics are live bacteria that are good for gut health. They may help to reduce the risk of intestinal damage and infection, and they may also boost the immune system.

- Vitamin D: Vitamin D is important for bone health, immune function, and cell growth. Many cancer patients are deficient in vitamin D, so it is important to supplement with it.

- Turmeric: Turmeric is a spice that contains curcumin, a compound with powerful anti-inflammatory and antioxidant properties. Curcumin has been shown to have anti-cancer effects in a number of studies.

- Resveratrol: Resveratrol is a compound found in red wine and grapes. It has anti-inflammatory, anti-oxidant, and anti-cancer properties.

It is important to note that there is limited research on the safety and efficacy of many nutritional supplements for cancer patients specifically. It is important to talk to your doctor before starting any new supplements, especially if you are taking any prescription medications.

HOW MUCH OF EACH SUPPLEMENT SHOULD BE TAKEN?

The dosage of each supplement will vary depending on the individual's needs. It is important to talk to your doctor to determine the right dosage for you.

Some general guidelines for the following supplements include:

- MCT oil: 1-2 tablespoons per day

- Omega-3 fatty acids: 1-2 grams per day

- Glutamine: 5-10 grams per day

- Electrolytes: Sodium: 2,300-3,000 milligrams per day, potassium: 2,000-3,500 milligrams per day, magnesium: 400-800 milligrams per day

- Multivitamin: Take a multivitamin that is specifically designed for cancer patients.

WHERE TO PURCHASE HIGH-QUALITY NUTRITIONAL SUPPLEMENTS

It is important to purchase high-quality nutritional supplements from a reputable retailer. Some good places to buy supplements include:

- Health food stores

- Online retailers, such as Amazon or iHerb

- Your doctor's office

When choosing supplements, be sure to read the label carefully and choose products that are third-party tested for purity and quality.

Nutritional supplements can be beneficial for cancer patients on the ketogenic diet. However, it is important to talk to your doctor before starting any new supplements, especially if you are taking any prescription medications.

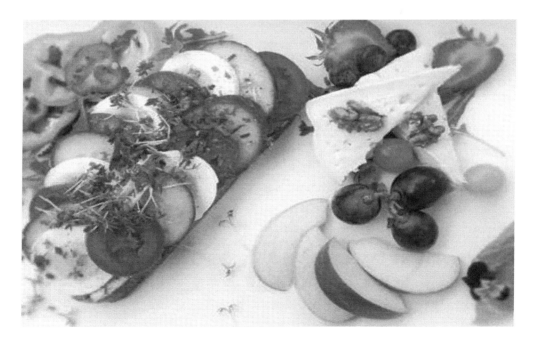

OTHER HEALTH CHALLENGES AND KETO

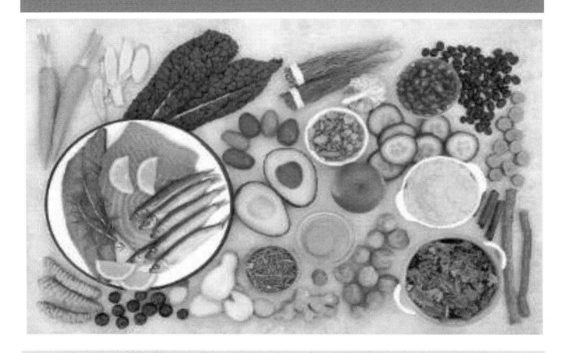

MANAGING DIABETES ON THE KETOGENIC DIET

The ketogenic diet can be a very effective way to manage diabetes, type 2 diabetes in particular. By restricting carbohydrates and focusing on healthy fats, the keto diet can help to lower blood sugar levels, improve insulin sensitivity, and reduce the risk of complications from diabetes.

However, it is important to note that the keto diet is not a magic bullet for diabetes management. It is important to work with your doctor to develop a personalized plan that is safe and effective for you.

Here are a few tips for managing diabetes on the ketogenic diet:

- Monitor your blood sugar levels regularly. This will help you to track your progress and make adjustments to your diet as needed.

- Be careful with your insulin dosage. As your blood sugar levels improve, you may need to reduce your insulin dosage. Talk to your doctor about how to adjust your insulin safely.

- Eat plenty of non-starchy vegetables. Vegetables are low in carbohydrates and high in nutrients, making them ideal for people on the keto diet.

- Choose healthy fats. Good sources of healthy fats include avocados, nuts, seeds, and olive oil.

- Avoid processed foods and sugary drinks. These foods are high in carbohydrates and can spike your blood sugar levels.

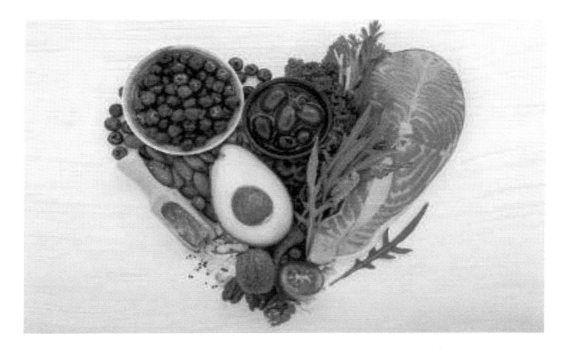

MANAGING HEART DISEASE ON THE KETOGENIC DIET

The ketogenic diet may also be beneficial for people with heart disease. Studies have shown that the keto diet can help to lower cholesterol levels, improve blood pressure, and reduce inflammation.

However, it is important to note that the keto diet is not without its risks. For example, the keto diet can increase the risk of kidney stones and gallstones. It is also important to monitor your electrolyte levels carefully, as the keto diet can deplete your body of electrolytes such as sodium and potassium.

If you have heart disease, it is important to talk to your doctor before starting the keto diet. Your doctor can help you to assess the risks and benefits of the diet for you and develop a personalized plan that is safe and effective.

MANAGING HIGH BLOOD PRESSURE ON THE KETOGENIC DIET

The ketogenic diet may also be helpful for people with high blood pressure. Studies have shown that the keto diet can help to lower blood pressure levels, especially in people with high blood pressure and obesity.

However, it is important to note that the keto diet is not without its risks. For example, the keto diet can increase the risk of kidney stones and gallstones. It is also important to monitor your electrolyte levels carefully, as the keto diet can deplete your body of electrolytes such as sodium and potassium.

If you have high blood pressure, it is important to talk to your doctor before starting the keto diet. Your doctor can help you to assess the risks and benefits of the diet for you and develop a personalized plan that is safe and effective.

MANAGING OTHER CHRONIC HEALTH CONDITIONS ON THE KETOGENIC DIET

The ketogenic diet may also be beneficial for people with other chronic health conditions, such as Alzheimer's disease, Parkinson's disease, and epilepsy. However, more research is needed to confirm these benefits.

If you have a chronic health condition, it is important to talk to your doctor before starting the keto diet. Your doctor can help you to assess the risks and benefits of the diet for you and develop a personalized plan that is safe and effective.

The ketogenic diet can be a safe and effective way to manage a variety of health conditions, including diabetes, heart disease, high blood pressure, and other chronic health conditions. However, it is important to talk to your doctor before starting the keto diet, especially if you have any underlying health conditions.

Your doctor can help you to assess the risks and benefits of the diet for you and develop a personalized plan that is safe and effective.

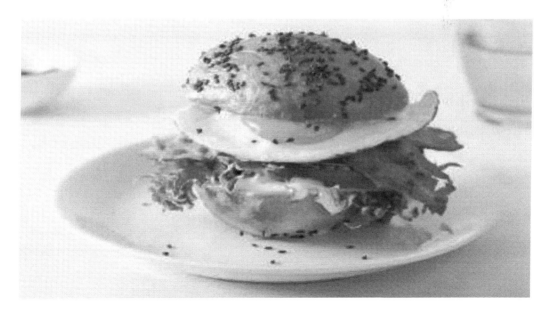

EVALUATING YOUR RESPONSE TO TREATMENT

Once you have started following the ketogenic diet for cancer, it is important to evaluate your response to treatment on a regular basis. This will help you to determine if the diet is working for you and to make any necessary adjustments.

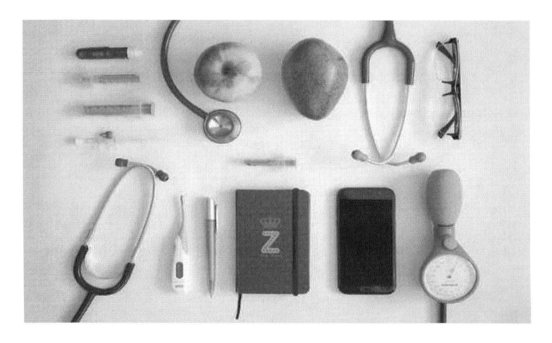

TRACKING YOUR PROGRESS

There are a number of ways to track your progress on the ketogenic diet. One way is to simply keep a journal of what you eat and how you feel each day. This will help you to identify any patterns or trends. You can also track your weight, body composition, and blood sugar levels.

Here are some specific things you may want to track:

- Weight: Weigh yourself at the same time each day, preferably before breakfast.

- Body composition: You can use a body composition scale to track your percentage of body fat, muscle mass, and water weight.

- Blood sugar levels: If you have diabetes, you will need to track your blood sugar levels regularly to make sure that the ketogenic diet is not causing them to go too high or too low.

COMMUNICATING WITH YOUR DOCTOR

It is important to communicate with your doctor on a regular basis while you are following the ketogenic diet for cancer. This will help to ensure that you are safe and that you are getting the most out of the diet.

Be sure to let your doctor know about any changes in your symptoms, weight, or blood sugar levels. You should also let them know about any new medications you are taking.

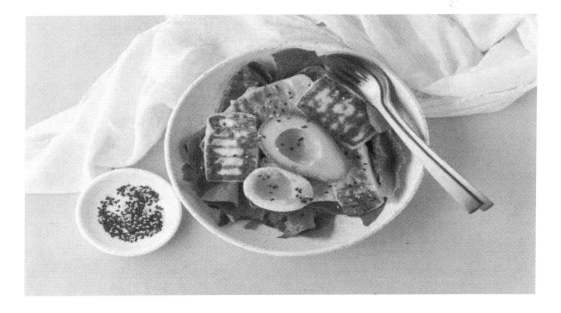

MAKING ADJUSTMENTS TO YOUR DIET AS NEEDED

If you are not seeing results with the ketogenic diet, or if you are experiencing any side effects, you may need to make some adjustments to your diet. You can talk to your doctor or a registered dietitian to get help with this.

Here are some common adjustments that may be needed:

- Increasing your carbohydrate intake: If you are not losing weight, you may need to increase your carbohydrate intake slightly. This will help to boost your metabolism and promote weight loss.

- Reducing your fat intake: If you are experiencing any side effects, such as nausea or diarrhea, you may need to reduce your fat intake.

- Adding more protein to your diet: Protein is essential for building and repairing muscle tissue. If you are not getting enough protein, you may experience muscle loss.

- Taking nutritional supplements: There are a number of nutritional supplements that can be beneficial for cancer patients on the ketogenic diet. Talk to your doctor about which supplements are right for you.

Evaluating your response to treatment on the ketogenic diet is important for ensuring that you are safe and that you are getting the most out of the diet. Track your progress, communicate with your doctor, and make adjustments to your diet as needed.

CONCLUSION

The ketogenic diet is a promising new approach to cancer treatment. While more research is needed, the existing evidence suggests that it can help to improve tumor response, reduce side effects, and improve quality of life.

If you are a cancer patient considering trying the ketogenic diet, it is important to talk to your doctor first. They can help you to determine if the ketogenic diet is right for you and to develop a safe and effective plan.

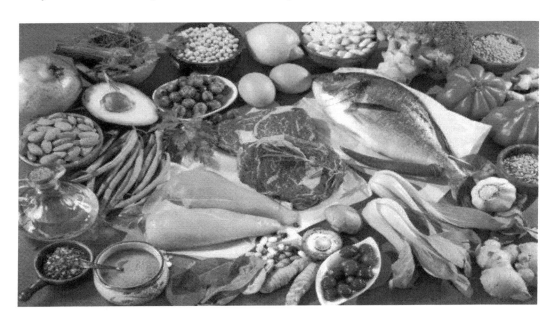

RESOURCES FOR CANCER PATIENTS ON THE KETOGENIC DIET

Here are some resources that can be helpful for cancer patients on the ketogenic diet:

- Cancer Nutrition Consulting Center: This organization provides free consultations with registered dietitians who specialize in the ketogenic diet for cancer patients.

- KetoCancer.org: This website provides a wealth of information on the ketogenic diet for cancer patients, including recipes, meal plans, and support groups.

INSPIRATIONAL STORIES FROM CANCER PATIENTS WHO HAVE BENEFITED FROM THE KETOGENIC DIET

Here are a few inspirational stories from cancer patients who have benefited from the ketogenic diet:

- Tricia Hersey: Tricia Hersey was diagnosed with stage 4 glioblastoma, a type of brain cancer, in 2017. She was given just six months to live. However, she decided to try the ketogenic diet, and it has been working wonders for her. She is now over five years in remission and is living a full and active life.

- Nick Cordero: Nick Cordero was a Broadway actor who was diagnosed with COVID-19 in 2020. He developed a number of complications, including a blood clot that cut off the blood supply to his leg. He had to have his leg amputated, and he also spent several months in a coma. While in the coma, he was put on the ketogenic diet. He eventually woke up from the coma, and he credits the ketogenic diet with helping him to recover.

- Terry Wahls: Terry Wahls was diagnosed with multiple sclerosis in 2000. She was slowly losing her ability to walk and talk. However, she decided to try the ketogenic diet, and it has transformed her life. She is now able to walk and talk again, and she is even able to run and exercise.

These are just a few examples of the many cancer patients who have benefited from the ketogenic diet. If you are a cancer patient considering trying the ketogenic diet, these stories should give you hope.

It is important to note that the ketogenic diet is not a cure for cancer. However, it can be a valuable tool for cancer patients who are looking to improve their quality of life and extend their survival time.

BONUS

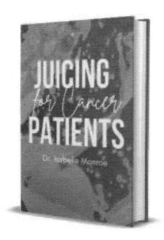

Scan the below QR code to Access A free Ebook

"Juicing for Cancer Patients"